Neonatal Care - Integrating Research With Clinical Practice

Edited by Seda Yilmaz Semerci

Published in London, United Kingdom

Neonatal Care - Integrating Research With Clinical Practice
http://dx.doi.org/10.5772/intechopen.1005945
Edited by Seda Yilmaz Semerci

Contributors
Adilova Aytakin, Aynur Polukhova, Donald R. Laub Jr, Dragan Katanić, Duygu Acar, Erhan Aygün, Genesis Carolina Vargas-Párraga, Genesis Leonor Miranda-Ordóñez, Giomar Rebeca Viteri-Gómez, Gulnara Mammadzada, Hossam A. Elgnainy, Ivett Beatriz Herrera-Quinde, Iyabode Olabisi Florence Dedeke, Javier Aquiles Hidalgo-Acosta, Maria Belen Herrera-Pinto, Mariam Rzayeva, María Fernanda Calderón León, Ming Yi, Naila Sultanova, Nushaba Panahova, Olatunbosun Oladipupo Olawale, Paula Elizabeth Pachucho-Hernández, Pusta Orujova, Seda Yilmaz Semerci, Sevda Quliyeva, Sheuli Chowdhury, Smelyng Francisco Sarango-Bravo, Tinuade Adetutu Ogunlesi, Tongyan Han, Victor Ayodeji Ayeni, Xinrui Huang

First published in London, United Kingdom, 2025 by IntechOpen
IntechOpen is the global imprint of INTECHOPEN LIMITED, registered in England and Wales, registration number: 11086078, 167-169 Great Portland Street, London, W1W 5PF, United Kingdom

For EU product safety concerns: IN TECH d.o.o., Prolaz Marije Krucifikse Kozulić 3, 51000 Rijeka, Croatia, info@intechopen.com or visit our website at intechopen.com.

British Library Cataloguing-in-Publication Data
A catalogue record for this book is available from the British Library

Neonatal Care - Integrating Research With Clinical Practice
Edited by Seda Yilmaz Semerci
p. cm.
Print ISBN 978-1-83634-635-7
Online ISBN 978-1-83634-634-0
eBook (PDF) ISBN 978-1-83634-636-4

If disposing of this product, please recycle the paper responsibly.

Meet the editor

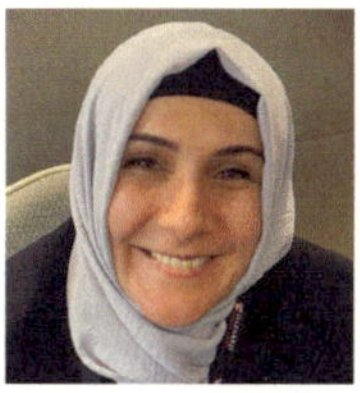

Seda Yilmaz Semerci is an Associate Professor, MD pediatrician and neonatologist based in Istanbul, Turkiye. A valedictorian graduate of Istanbul University, she completed advanced training at leading institutions, including Harvard Medical School and the Max Planck Institute. Dr. Yilmaz Semerci has authored over 40 peer-reviewed articles, contributed to multiple international books and projects on neonatology. She has received numerous awards and serves as Editor-in-Chief of the Journal of Child Science. Renowned for her research in neonatal intensive care, bioinformatics, and medical education, she is committed to advancing newborn care both in Turkiye and internationally. Outside of medicine, she enjoys calligraphy and photography.

Contents

Preface

In the field of pediatric medicine, neonatology has a pivotal role, where advancements in research and clinical practice have a direct influence on the very beginning of the lives of our most vulnerable patients. As we delve into the complexities of neonatal health, we aim to illuminate the recent advancements that continue to shape our understanding and management of neonatal conditions. This book provides a comprehensive examination of key topics, including the fundamentals of neonatal sepsis, parenteral nutrition, neonatal endocrine disorders, and other relevant areas. Each section will address recent advancements, including the application of artificial intelligence in assessing the general movements of newborn infants, novel therapeutic agents for hypoxic-ischemic encephalopathy, neonatal seizures, and effects of anesthesia during the neonatal period.

As we navigate these essential topics, we seek to emphasize the integration of innovative technologies and therapies that enhance neonatal care.

The combination of rigorous research and clinical application will empower healthcare professionals to make informed decisions, thereby enriching our collective efforts to improve neonatal health.

Thank you for your efforts in this essential discourse as we strive to advance knowledge and practice in the field of neonatology, benefiting our most precious patients.

Best regards,

Seda Yilmaz Semerci
Istinye University,
School of Medicine,
Istanbul, Turkiye

Chapter 1

Sepsis in the Neonatal Period

Javier Aquiles Hidalgo-Acosta,
Genesis Carolina Vargas-Párraga, Ivett Beatriz Herrera-Quinde,
Maria Belen Herrera-Pinto, Smelyng Francisco Sarango-Bravo,
Genesis Leonor Miranda-Ordóñez,
Paula Elizabeth Pachucho-Hernández,
Giomar Rebeca Viteri-Gómez
and María Fernanda Calderón León

Abstract

Neonatal sepsis is one of the main causes of mortality in premature newborns worldwide; the infection can be acquired during pregnancy, childbirth, or during hospital admission to the neonatal intensive care unit. Mortality from sepsis increases considerably with the appearance of antibiotic-resistant germs. Neonatal sepsis is one of the main causes of morbidity and mortality in preterm infants worldwide. Special care should be taken in prenatal control with genitourinary tract infections to avoid premature rupture of membranes with bacterial ascent complicated by chorioamnionitis, also considering that the administration of intrapartum antibiotics has not been shown to reduce mortality from neonatal sepsis. The use of penicillin plus gentamicin is one of the best schemes, with less effects on bacterial resistance and translocation. The most common germs in neonatal-onset sepsis include group B *Streptococcus*, *Escherichia coli*, *Klebsiella pneumoniae*, *Staphylococcus aureus*, *Enterococcus* sp., coagulase-negative *Staphylococcus*, *Streptococcus agalactiae*, and *Serratia marcescens*. Neonatal invasive candidiasis is a common cause of invasive fungal disease in low-birth-weight preterm infants. The viruses are associated with necrotizing enterocolitis, myocarditis, and respiratory failure.

Keywords: neonatal intensive care units, neonatal sepsis, critical care, pregnancy complications, infectious diseases

1. Introduction

This chapter is highly relevant due to the need to adequately manage neonatal bacterial, fungal, or viral sepsis that can progressively invade and cause organ failure; therefore, it is important to know how to recognize it early to avoid its progression to multi-organ failure with high mortality in the neonatal intensive care unit.

Neonatal sepsis is defined as a state of multisystem dysfunction in the newborn, secondary to an infection that causes organ failure of the following types: neurological, respiratory, cardiovascular, hematological, digestive, renal, or metabolic [1].

Septic shock is an alteration of homeostasis, a product of infection that causes acute circulatory failure, due to the patient's unregulated response to the infection and is characterized by hypotension and hypoperfusion requiring treatment with vasopressors and mechanical ventilation [2].

Classification of infections in the neonate is useful as a guide to the possible causative agent of the infection to which empirical treatment is directed [3]. Neonatal infections can be classified: (1) according to the time of onset of signs and symptoms of infection; (2) by the time of contagion; (3) according to the origin of the infection; and (4) based on the mode of transmission [4].

Neonatal sepsis according to its onset can be classified into two traditional types: early-onset neonatal sepsis, when the infection originates in the first 72 hours after delivery, and late-onset neonatal sepsis, which occurs from 72 hours of life to 28 days after delivery [5].

According to the time of infection, it can be classified as: prenatal sepsis secondary to infections of pregnancy, the placenta, amniotic fluid, and membranes. Sepsis due to infection with natal is transmitted during delivery, and postnatal sepsis is acquired during the neonatal period [6].

Based on the origin, neonatal sepsis is divided into perinatal, community-acquired, and health care-associated or nosocomial sepsis [7].

Depending on the mode of transmission, neonatal infections can be vertically transmitted or horizontally transmitted. Vertical infection occurs during pregnancy, childbirth, or breastfeeding, and horizontal transmission refers to infections in the community or associated with healthcare.

Sepsis is a common pathology in neonatology, being one of the main causes of mortality in premature babies, mainly those with very low birth weight, whose infection can be acquired during pregnancy, childbirth, or during hospital admission; its etiology is variable, as shown in **Table 1** [20].

Mortality ranges from 11 to 19% [8, 21] and can reach up to 29% in very low-birth-weight premature infants [22]. Neonatal sepsis is an important cause of neonatal mortality. The most frequent complications include perinatal asphyxia, intrauterine fetal distress, contamination by meconium fluid (**Figures 1** and **2**), lower for gestational age, perinatal fever, and very low birth weight in the neonatal intensive care unit [23].

Risk factors for neonatal sepsis are: prematurity, low birth weight, chorioamnionitis, premature rupture of membranes, low APGAR, inability to breastfeed, prolonged hospital stay, and invasive procedures, as shown in **Figure 1**. The birth of a newborn in cephalic presentation with membranes and amniotic fluid with the presence of meconium is observed in **Figure 2**; a newborn with fetal malformation (gastroschisis) is observed who later presented neonatal sepsis and required NICU [1].

Diagnosis with special techniques, such as molecular methods and mass spectrometry, has been shown to be an alternative to cultures; however, blood cultures remain the diagnostic standard [24]. NICE guidelines divide risk factors into indicators and use laboratory tests for clinical decision-making and determining the duration of treatment [25]. Biomarkers such as C-reactive protein, procalcitonin, and serum amyloid A are useful for the early diagnosis of neonatal sepsis [26].

Bacterial	Fungal	Viral
Group B *streptococcus* (SGB) and *Escherichia coli* are the most common pathogens in early-onset sepsis. Gram-negative germs such as *Klebsiella pneumoniae*, Gram-positive Staphylococcus aureus, *Enterococcus* spn, coagulase-negative *Staphylococcus*, *Streptococcus agalactiae*, *Serratia marcescens*. Multi-resistant bacteria, the agents of nosocomial infections *Acinetobacter* spp., *Klebsiella* spp. *Escherichia coli* can cause keratitis, conjunctivitis, urinary tract infections, pneumonia, surgical wound infections, bacteremia, and meningitis in the neonatal intensive care unit. The germs with the highest multi-resistance are: *Acinetobacter* spp., *Klebsiella* spp., and *Escherichia coli* [9–11].	Neonatal invasive candidiasis is the most frequent cause of invasive fungal disease in premature low-birth-weight newborns; for this reason, it is necessary to start empirical treatment early [12]. Diagnosis requires high suspicion accompanied by a test such as positive blood culture; beta-D-glucan is detected in the presence of invasive mycoses such as Aspergillosis, Fusariosis, Candidiasis, Pneumocystosis, and Cryptococcosis [13–15].	Rotavirus and norovirus are associated with necrotizing enterocolitis, increasing the risk in newborns. Severe neonatal enterovirus infection has a high mortality rate, as it can cause myocarditis requiring mechanical ventilation and extracorporeal membrane oxygenation, which represents a high risk of mortality in the neonatal intensive care unit [16–18]. Respiratory syncytial virus, herpes simplex virus, and enterovirus are frequent causes of neonatal sepsis, and additional studies such as PCR tests are needed for diagnosis [19].

Table 1.
Etiology of neonatal sepsis, most frequent microorganisms [6–8].

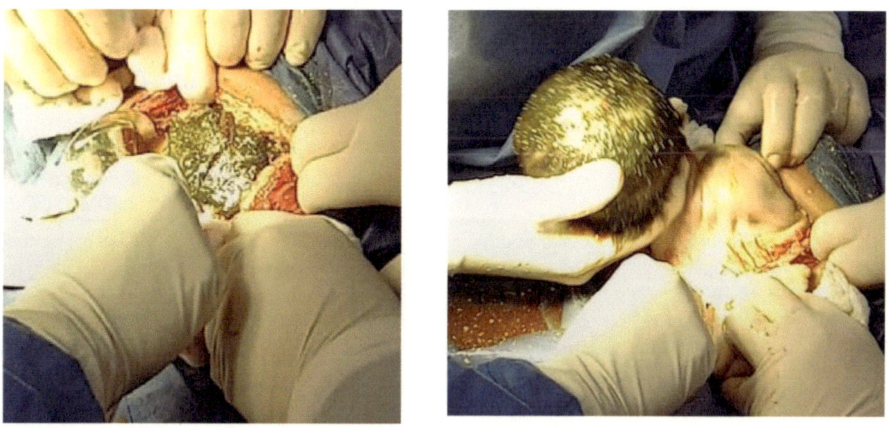

Figure 1.
Image 1 of a newborn born in a cephalic presentation with membranes and amniotic fluid stained with the presence of meconium.

Clinical signs, complemented by positive cultures, provide the diagnosis of sepsis [27]. Etiologically, it is caused by multiple germs as observed in **Tables 1** and **2**. When traditional cultures do not report a germ, it is necessary to perform polymerase chain reaction studies.

Early neonatal sepsis, which occurs in the first 72 hours of the neonatal period, is associated with pregnancy infections, for example, chorioamnionitis [31]. Late sepsis occurs more than 72 hours after delivery [32].

Diagnostic interventions include: lumbar puncture, urine culture, blood culture, bronchial secretion culture, and stool culture, which are necessary in the

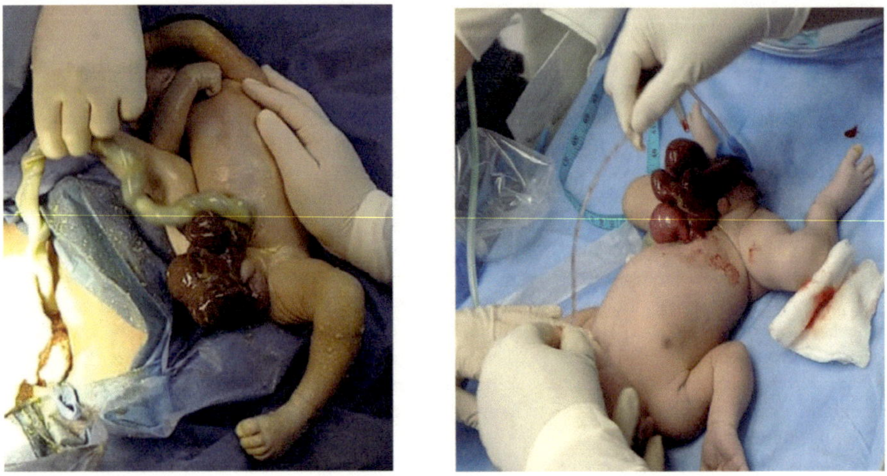

Figure 2.
Image 2 of a newborn with fetal malformation (gastroschisis) delivered by cesarean section and diagnosed with neonatal sepsis.

Author	Multi-resistance	Etiologic agent	Endurance	Results
Wattal C, Kler N, Oberoi J, et al.	Neonatal sepsis due to multidrug-resistance (MDR)	*Klebsiella pneumonia, E. coli and Acinetobacter baumannii, E. cloacae, Burkholderia cepacia, Pseudomonas aeruginosa*	Cefotaxime (87%), ciprofloxacin (70%), and trimethoprim/ sulfamethoxazole (76%).	87% extended β-lactamase (ESBL)-producing isolates, 6% metallo β-lactamase (MBL)-producing isolates, meropenem-resistant New Delhi metallo β-lactamase-1 (NDM-1) isolates
Mutlu, M., Aslan, Y., Aktürk Acar, et al.	Microbiological profile and antibiotic susceptibility of germs isolated in cultures in neonatal nosocomial sepsis	Gram-positive, Gram-negative, and fungal, coagulase-negative *staphylococci* (CoNS), *Klebsiella* pneumoniae, and *C. guilliermondii*.	Oxacillin-resistant CoNS strains and extended-spectrum beta-lactamase (ESBL)-producing strains.	Low susceptibility to antibiotics commonly used for empirical treatment in neonatal sepsis.
Lutsar I, Chazallon C, Trafojer U, et al.	Meropenem versus standard therapy for late-onset neonatal sepsis (NeoMero1):	Gram-positive, Gram-negative, and mixed, acquisition of meropenem-resistant Gram-negative bacteria occurred in 4% of the meropenem group and 12% of the standard treatment group ($p = 0.052$).	Standard treatment (Ampicillin+gentamicin or cefotaxime+gentamicin) chosen by each center before the start of the study for 8–14 days.	Successful outcome (32%) in the meropenem group versus (23%) in the standard treatment group ($p = 0.087$).

Table 2.
Most common bacteria that generate bacterial resistance to multiple antibiotics [28–30].

management of neonatal sepsis, mainly cultures, which are highly important because they allow the identification of the germ, in addition to providing targeted treatment with a beneficial effect that improves the results and, thus, access to knowledge of antibiotic sensitivity, which is essential. Rapid diagnostic techniques such as fluorescent *in situ* hybridization can also be applied, which together with culture are the gold standard in the diagnosis of neonatal sepsis [33].

An advance in diagnosis includes biomarkers in sepsis, accompanied by modern detection techniques that identify early the etiology of neonatal sepsis [34]. Among the main associated biomarkers are serum amyloid A, C-reactive protein, procalcitonin, and lipopolysaccharide binding protein [35]; other biomarkers and additional tests are useful in fungal sepsis due to invasive mycoses such as galactomannan, germ tube antibody for *Candida albicans*, 1,3-β-d-glucan, polymerase chain reaction, and T2 Candida panel. Echocardiogram is useful when candidiasis is suspected, showing the presence of vegetations on the valves or central catheters. The use of ophthalmoscopy is also very beneficial to visualize ocular infection in patients with invasive candidiasis, which improves the performance of treatment [9].

2. Prognostic scales

The nSOFA is a sequential neonatal organ failure assessment that estimates the risk of mortality based on the number of organs with multi-organ failure. The nSOFA score allows us to predict mortality. A value nSOFA > 4 will result in a higher mortality rate of 67% compared to neonates with an nSOFA < 4, resulting in a mortality rate of 13% ($p < 0.001$). Mortality increases by the hour as the nSOFA remains elevated [36].

Among the prognostic scales, there are: the NOSEP-1 scale, which uses five clinical and laboratory parameters that contain: C-reactive protein, neutrophils, platelets, parenteral nutrition, and fever. The scales NOSEP 2, NOSEP NEW I, and NOSEP-NEW-II incorporate recent surgery, maternal hypertension, ventilation, and heart rate characteristic index; these scales are used to evaluate neonatal sepsis through the mentioned parameters [37].

Mortality from neonatal sepsis is variable as shown in **Table 3**, depending on the region of study, being lower in more developed countries. The percentages vary

Mortality due to neonatal sepsis	Statistics by region (country)
19.70%	Ghana NICU
18.40%	NICU of Brazil
15%	NICU of the United States of America
Multidrug-resistant (MR) patients had 60% mortality versus 13% non-MR	Jordan NICU
Mortality in patients treated with meropenem in late sepsis was: 6% overall and 10% in Gram-negative sepsis.	NICUs from six countries

Mortality ranges from 15 to 18.4%, which increases due to multi-resistant germs; mortality can reach up to 60% in cases of bacterial multi-resistance [28, 29, 38–40].

Table 3.
Mortality of neonatal sepsis according to demographic region.

between 19.70% for the neonatal ICUs of Ghana, 18.40% in neonatal ICUs of Brazil, and 15% mortality in the United States of America, Europe, and Asia; as resistance increases, mortality increases [28, 29, 38–40].

3. Methodology

By inclusion and exclusion, published articles on the research topic with available results were selected. Inclusion criteria were articles on neonatal sepsis and its management, neonatal sepsis in the intensive care unit, strategies for the management of early and late neonatal sepsis, and mortality from neonatal sepsis in the NICU. Inconclusive articles without results that did not address the research topic were excluded. The articles were obtained from databases such as the National Library of Medicine, PubMed, Elsevier, Europe PMC, X-MOL, National Certification Corporation, and journals such as: Current International Guidelines on neonatal sepsis, Nature, BMJ, JAMA, and New England Journal of Medicine, consulted with the last search date February 11, 2025.

4. Start and duration of treatment

It is important to recognize the golden hour of sepsis, which is the ideal time to start treatment from the moment neonatal sepsis is recognized, which is focused on maintaining treatment empirically until obtaining the results of the cultures. However, cultures do not have a specificity and sensitivity of 100%; therefore, the decision of the duration of treatment cannot be made entirely based on the result. The treatment time will depend on the clinical suspicion and characteristics of the patient, as well as additional tests [41].

As seen in **Table 4**, the duration of antibiotic treatment for neonatal sepsis of bacterial origin can be maintained from 8 to 14 days.

After a diagnosis with a positive culture for a mycosis, it is necessary to monitor blood cultures until they are negative, and it is recommended to continue treatment for 14 days after the negative result, especially in cases of invasive mycoses [50].

Intrapartum antibiotic administration has not been shown to decrease mortality from neonatal sepsis [36, 42]. The use of penicillin plus gentamicin is one of the best regimens, with less effects on resistance and bacterial translocation, in contrast to the use of amoxicillin plus cefotaxime [37, 43]. Another study also maintains evidence that antibiotic therapy with ampicillin plus gentamicin is a standard empirical regimen for the management of neonatal sepsis compared to other drugs such as fosfomycin [38, 44]. Other therapies include cefotaxime and vancomycin, while broad-spectrum regimens will be reserved for antibiotic-resistant germs [28, 39, 40, 45, 46, 51].

The duration of antibiotic treatment with positive culture and good therapeutic response should be maintained for 10 days since longer duration regimens have not shown any benefit (**Table 4**) [29, 41, 47, 52]. In addition, adjuvant therapy to antibiotic treatment with vitamin D is necessary, since decreased levels have been observed in patients with neonatal sepsis [50, 53], as well as the supplementation of trace elements such as zinc, which has been shown to be effective in the management of late sepsis [42, 54].

Author	Intervention	Treatment	Results
Roca A, et al. [42]	Intrapartum azithromycin vs. placebo	1:1 ratio during labor.	Incidence of neonatal mortality or sepsis was similar in both groups
Reyman M, et al. [43]	Evaluation of antibiotic effects on the intestinal flora of infants	Three therapeutic options were used: 1. Penicillin + gentamicin 2. Amoxicillin plus clavulanic acid + gentamicin 3. Amoxicillin + cefotaxime	Amoxicillin + cefotaxime had the greatest effects on the genetic profile of antibiotic resistance; penicillin + gentamicin had the least effects.
Reddy A, et al. [47]	Evaluation of the duration of antibiotic treatment in culture-proven neonatal sepsis	Neonates with sepsis were randomly assigned to 10 days of antibiotic therapy, and another group received antibiotic therapy for 14 days.	Antibiotic treatment has achieved clinical and microbiological remission on day 7 compared to longer regimens.
Obiero CW, et al. [44]	Use of fosfomycin in neonatal sepsis	They compared ampicillin and gentamicin versus intravenous fosfomycin at 150 mg/kg twice daily and then orally at 100 mg/kg twice daily for up to 7 days.	Fosfomycin offers potential utility as a regimen with a simple dosing schedule for neonatal sepsis.
Zhang F, [45]	Efficacy of cefotaxime combined with gamma globulins on C-reactive protein and procalcitonin in neonatal sepsis	Children in the control group were treated with cefotaxime, while children in the observation group were treated with cefotaxime combined with gamma globulins.	Cefotaxime combined with gamma globulin in the treatment of neonatal sepsis has significant efficacy and is clinically more effective than cefotaxime monotherapy.
Xu YB, et al. [46].	Effects of vancomycin and cefotaxime combined with gamma globulin, respectively, in neonatal sepsis and their influences on PCT and CRP	Vancomycin and cefotaxime combined with gamma globulin, respectively, in neonatal sepsis	Vancomycin combined with gamma globulin were selected as group A (96 cases). and those treated with cefotaxime combined with gamma globulin were selected as group B (85 cases). Hospital stay in group A was shorter than in group B ($p < 0.05$), drug effects in group B was better than in group A ($p < 0.05$).
Lutsar I, et al. [29]	Meropenem versus standard therapy for the management of late-onset neonatal sepsis (NeoMero1):	Randomized in a 1:1 ratio to receive meropenem versus standard treatment (ampicillin + gentamicin or cefotaxime + gentamicin) chosen by each site prior to study entry for 8–14 days.	Successful outcome (32%) in the meropenem group versus (23%) in the standard treatment group ($p = 0.087$).
Kim J, et al. [48]	Caspofungin versus amphotericin B deoxycholate in the treatment of invasive candidiasis in neonates	2 mg/kg caspofungin intravenously once daily or 1 mg/kg amphotericin B deoxycholate	The survival rate at 2 weeks after treatment was 71.0% in the caspofungin group and 68.8% in the amphotericin group. Amphotericin had more adverse effects with similar mortality.

Author	Intervention	Treatment	Results
Auriti C, et al. [49]	High-dose micafungin in neonates and young infants with invasive candidiasis	Micafungin at a dose of 8 mg/kg	Resolution of the infection was achieved in 86.7% of treated patients. Micafungin at a dose of 8 mg/kg daily is effective and well tolerated in neonates and infants.

Table 4.
Summary of clinical trials evaluating the treatment of neonatal sepsis of bacterial and fungal origin [29, 42–49].

Intravenous fluconazole has been effective with good results in premature neonates. Other therapeutic options include the use of echinocandins such as caspofungin, anidulafungin, or micafungin, which have been beneficial in fungal sepsis [43–46, 55–58]. In cases of invasive candidiasis, amphotericin B achieves recovery and resolution of the infection with good results, as evidenced in clinical studies on different available treatments (**Table 4**) [48, 49, 51, 52].

5. Discussion

The results of the review emphasize the need to provide early treatment when sepsis is clinically recognized and with the help of new biomarkers for diagnosis, treatment, and follow-up.

The importance and usefulness of molecular tests to recognize the causative agent of the infection is described.

The vast majority of clinical studies analyzed used early and late classification to evaluate diagnosis and treatment.

Another important point is intrapartum antibiotics; no evidence was found to support that their routine use reduces neonatal sepsis, because in many cases the infection is already established in the newborn, even during pregnancy.

A study was found showing that azithromycin administered as a neonatal sepsis prevention strategy does not reduce mortality compared to placebo.

Neonatal sepsis guidelines recognize the classification of early and late sepsis as the most commonly used and that laboratory diagnostic tests are not sensitive or specific enough to decide on management alone and should be associated with the patient's clinical response [59].

Although intrapartum antibiotics are widely used in the context of preventing puerperal sepsis, their use is justified, for example, in cases such as chorioamnionitis with prolonged rupture of membranes, where there are high rates of risk of neonatal sepsis, although the maternal benefit is greater than the neonatal benefit [60].

There is insufficient evidence to justify antibiotic prophylaxis in a pregnant woman who is pregnant at term and has premature rupture of membranes (PROM) in less than 24 hours, except in the case of patients with GBS. In cases of PROM <24 hours and negative GBS, antibiotic therapy is not started coinciding with the end of pregnancy [61].

Only if the patient presents uterine dynamics + positive GBS + PROM + full-term pregnancy, will we administer ATB upon admission with the following therapeutic options: (1) Penicillin 5 M intravenous initial dose and then penicillin 2.5 M/4 h intravenous or (2) ampicillin 2 g intravenous initial dose and then 1 g/4 h intravenous. If the patient does not have uterine activity, (3) Amoxicillin/clavulanic acid 1 g/6 hours intravenously can be used. In cases of allergies, administer: Clindamycin 900 mg/8 h intravenous. If there is resistance to clindamycin, it is recommended to use teicoplanin 600 mg/24 h intravenously [61].

In pregnant women with PPROM of ≥24 hours of evolution, the plan consists of: additional tests including complete blood count and PCR. Antibiotic therapy: with amoxicillin-clavulanic acid 1 g/6 hours intravenously, regardless of the carrier status of GBS. In cases of allergy to beta-lactams, intravenous clindamycin is recommended. Termination of pregnancy: Termination of pregnancy will be scheduled upon admission [61].

PROM in preterm pregnancy: In these cases, broad-spectrum prophylactic antibiotic therapy will be started with ampicillin 2 g/6 h intravenously + ceftriaxone 1 g/12 h intravenously + clarithromycin 500 mg/12 h orally. The proposed antibiotic prophylaxis is broad-spectrum and has good safety for both the fetus and the mother [61].

In case of allergies to penicillin or beta-lactams: The prophylaxis of choice will be the combination of teicoplanin 600 mg/24 h intravenous + aztreonam 1 g/8 h intravenous + clarithromycin 500 mg/12 h orally [61].

If clinical chorioamnionitis is suspected, the pregnancy will be terminated under antibiotic coverage with piperacillin-tazobactam 4.5 g every 6 hours intravenously + clarithromycin 500 mg/12 orally. After vaginal delivery or cesarean delivery, the same antibiotic therapy will be maintained for 48 hours; unless the patient remains febrile after this period, antibiotic treatment will be continued for more than 48 hours. In these cases, the dose and type of drug will be individualized based on the results of the cultures [61].

6. Conclusions

The definition of neonatal sepsis depends on clinical criteria, laboratory tests, or the presence of positive cultures, with the initiation of early empirical antibiotic therapy in the first hour being of great importance.

Antibiotics represent the gold standard for the management of neonatal sepsis; however, other types of fungal infections such as invasive candidiasis also arise, requiring a high index of suspicion and initiation of antifungal therapy.

Cultures continue to be the most widely used standard for diagnosis, but the use of polymerase chain reaction or biomarkers for selected cases are new diagnostic trends that may improve future survival.

Since there is no highly specific and/or sensitive biomarker that indicates the early diagnosis of neonatal sepsis, the clinical evaluation and physical examination of the physician should be included as the cornerstone of the (early) diagnosis; the most commonly used biomarkers are CRP and procalcitonin, being more useful during patient monitoring in their therapeutic response.

Acknowledgements

Special thanks to Professor Juana Narcisa Acosta Alcívar for her unconditional support throughout my life.

Conflict of interest

The authors declare no conflict of interest.

Acronyms and abbreviations

NICU	neonatal intensive care unit

Author details

Javier Aquiles Hidalgo-Acosta[1*], Genesis Carolina Vargas-Párraga[2], Ivett Beatriz Herrera-Quinde[3], Maria Belen Herrera-Pinto[1], Smelyng Francisco Sarango-Bravo[4], Genesis Leonor Miranda-Ordóñez[5], Paula Elizabeth Pachucho-Hernández[1], Giomar Rebeca Viteri-Gómez[5] and María Fernanda Calderón León[6]

1 University of Guayaquil, Ecuador

2 Enrique Ortega Hospital, Duran, Ecuador

3 Mount Sinai Hospital, Guayaquil, Ecuador

4 Hospital University of Guayaquil, Ecuador

5 Catholic University of Santiago of Guayaquil, Ecuador

6 Catholic University of Guayaquil, Ecuador

*Address all correspondence to: jahidalgoacosta@hotmail.com

References

[1] Odabasi IO, Bulbul A. Neonatal sepsis. Sisli Etfal Hastanesi Tip Bulteni. 2020;**54**(2):142-158. DOI: 10.14744/SEMB.2020.00236

[2] McGovern M, Giannoni E, Kuester H, Turner MA, van den Hoogen A, Bliss JM, et al. Infection, inflammation, immunology and immunization (I4) section of the ESPR. Challenges in developing a consensus definition of neonatal sepsis. Pediatric Research. 2020;**88**(1):14-26. DOI: 10.1038/s41390-020-0785-x

[3] Russell N, Barday M, Okomo U, Dramowski A, Sharland M, Bekker A. Early-versus late-onset sepsis in neonates - Time to shift the paradigm? Clinical Microbiology and Infection. 2024;**30**(1):38-43. DOI: 10.1016/j.cmi.2023.07.023

[4] Mariani M, Parodi A, Minghetti D, Ramenghi LA, Palmero C, Ugolotti E, et al. Early and late onset neonatal sepsis: Epidemiology and effectiveness of empirical antibacterial therapy in a III level neonatal intensive care unit. Antibiotics (Basel). 2022;**11**(2):284. DOI: 10.3390/antibiotics11020284

[5] Harrison ML, Dickson BFR, Sharland M, Williams PCM. Beyond early- and late-onset neonatal sepsis definitions: What are the current causes of neonatal sepsis globally? A systematic review and meta-analysis of the evidence. The Pediatric Infectious Disease Journal. 2024;**43**(12):1182-1190. DOI: 10.1097/INF.0000000000004485

[6] Pace E, Yanowitz T. Infections in the NICU: Neonatal sepsis. Seminars in Pediatric Surgery. 2022;**31**(4):151200. DOI: 10.1016/j.semptsurg.2022.151200

[7] Manuel DÁ. Most common causal microorganisms and risk factors according to the classification of neonatal infections. Revista Cubana de Pediatría. 2021;**93**(2):1-20. Available from: http://scielo.sld.cu/scielo.php?script=sci_arttext&pid=S0034-75312021000200015&lng=es

[8] Flannery DD, Puopolo KM. Neonatal early-onset sepsis. NeoReviews. 2022;**23**(11):756-770. DOI: 10.1542/neo.23-10-e756

[9] Fleiss N, Polin RA. Sequential organ failure assessment scores to predict outcomes: From adults to neonates. Current Opinion in Pediatrics. 2023;**35**(2):218-222. DOI: 10.1097/MOP.0000000000001207

[10] Cristina ML, Sartini M, Spagnolo AM. Serratia marcescens infections in neonatal intensive care units (NICUs). International Journal of Environmental Research and Public Health. 2019;**16**(4):610. DOI: 10.3390/ijerph16040610

[11] Dudeja S. Neonatal sepsis: Treatment of neonatal sepsis in multidrug-resistant (MDR) infections: Part 2. Indian Journal of Pediatrics. 2020;**87**(2):122-124. DOI: 10.1007/s12098-019-03152-7

[12] Ferrando G, Castagnola E. Prophylaxis of invasive fungal infection in neonates: A narrative review for practical purposes. Journal of Fungi (Basel). 2023;**9**(2):164. DOI: 10.3390/jof9020164

[13] Cohen JF, Ouziel A, Matczak S, Brice J, Spijker R, Lortholary O, et al. Diagnostic accuracy of serum (1,3)-beta-d-glucan for neonatal invasive candidiasis: Systematic review and

meta-analysis. Clinical Microbiology and Infection. 2020;**26**(3):291-298. DOI: 10.1016/j.cmi.2019.09.010

[14] Georgescu TA, Lisievici AC, Munteanu O, Furtunescu FL, Bratu OG, Berceanu C, et al. Congenital systemic candidiasis: A comprehensive literature review and meta-analysis of 44 cases. Romanian Journal of Morphology and Embryology. 2020;**61**(3):673-680. DOI: 10.47162/RJME.61.3.05

[15] Ferreras-Antolin L, Aziz N, Warris A. Serial (1-3)-beta-D-Glucan (BDG) monitoring shows high variability among premature neonates. Medical Mycology. 2022;**60**(6):myac032. DOI: 10.1093/mmy/myac032

[16] Mani S, Hazra S, Hagan J, Sisson A, Nair J, Pammi M. Viral infections and neonatal necrotizing enterocolitis: A meta-analysis. Pediatrics. 2023;**152**(1):e2022060876. DOI: 10.1542/peds.2022-060876

[17] Zhang M, Wang H, Tang J, He Y, Xiong T, Li W, et al. Clinical characteristics of severe neonatal enterovirus infection: A systematic review. BMC Pediatrics. 2021;**21**(1):127. DOI: 10.1186/s12887-021-02599-y

[18] Cortina G, Best D, Deisenberg M, Chiletti R, Butt W. Extracorporeal membrane oxygenation for neonatal collapse caused by enterovirus myocarditis. Archives of Disease in Childhood-Fetal and Neonatal Edition. 2018;**103**(4):F370-F376. DOI: 10.1136/archdischild-2016-312429

[19] Dong Y, Basmaci R, Titomanlio L, Sun B, Mercier JC. Neonatal sepsis: Within and beyond China. Chinese Medical Journal. 2020;**133**(18):2219-2228. DOI: 10.1097/CM9.0000000000000935

[20] Bethou A, Bhat BV. Neonatal sepsis-newer insights. Indian Journal of Pediatrics. 2022;**89**(3):267-273. DOI: 10.1007/s12098-021-03852-z

[21] Molloy EJ, Bearer CF. Pediatric and neonatal sepsis and inflammation. Pediatric Research. 2022;**91**(2):267-269. DOI: 10.1038/s41390-021-01918-4

[22] Stoll BJ, Puopolo KM, Hansen NI, Sánchez PJ, Bell EF, Carlo WA, et al. Early-onset neonatal sepsis 2015 to 2017, the rise of *Escherichia coli*, and the need for novel prevention strategies. JAMA Pediatrics. 2020;**174**(7):e200593. DOI: 10.1001/jamapediatrics.2020.0593

[23] Guo L, Han W, Su Y, Wang N, Chen X, Ma J, et al. Perinatal risk factors for neonatal early-onset sepsis: A meta-analysis of observational studies. The Journal of Maternal-Fetal & Neonatal Medicine. 2023;**36**(2):2259049. DOI: 10.1080/14767058.2023.2259049

[24] Celik IH, Hanna M, Canpolat FE, Pammi M. Diagnosis of neonatal sepsis: The past, present and future. Pediatric Research. 2022;**91**(2):337-350. DOI: 10.1038/s41390-021-01696-z

[25] Balayan S, Chauhan N, Chandra R, Kuchhal NK, Jain U. Recent advances in developing biosensing based platforms for neonatal sepsis. Biosensors & Bioelectronics. 2020;**169**:112552. DOI: 10.1016/j.bios.2020.112552

[26] Gopal N, Chauhan N, Jain U, Dass SK, Sharma HS, Chandra R. Advancement in biomarker based effective diagnosis of neonatal sepsis. Artificial Cells, Nanomedicine, and Biotechnology. 2023;**51**(1):476-490. DOI: 10.1080/21691401.2023.2252016

[27] Hayes R, Hartnett J, Semova G, Murray C, Murphy K, Carroll L, et al. Neonatal sepsis definitions from

randomized clinical trials. Pediatric Research. 2023;**93**(5):1141-1148. DOI: 10.1038/s41390-021-01749-3

[28] Wattal C, Kler N, Oberoi JK, Fursule A, Kumar A, Thakur A. Neonatal sepsis: Mortality and morbidity in neonatal sepsis due to multidrug-resistant (MDR) organisms: Part 1. Indian Journal of Pediatrics. 2020;**87**(2):117-121. DOI: 10.1007/s12098-019-03106-z. Epub 2019 Dec 11. Erratum in: Indian J Pediatr. 2020 Oct;87(10):880. doi:10.1007/s12098-020-03256-5

[29] Lutsar I, Chazallon C, Trafojer U, de Cabre VM, Auriti C, Bertaina C, et al. Meropenem vs standard of care for treatment of neonatal late onset sepsis (NeoMero1): A randomized controlled trial. PLoS One. 2020;**15**(3):e0229380. DOI: 10.1371/journal.pone.0229380

[30] Mutlu M, Aslan Y, Aktürk Acar F, Kader Ş, Bayramoğlu G, Yılmaz G. Changing trend of microbiological profile and antibiotic susceptibility of the microorganisms isolated in the neonatal nosocomial sepsis: A 14 years analysis. The Journal of Maternal-Fetal & Neonatal Medicine. 2020;**33**(21):3658-3665. DOI: 10.1080/14767058.2019.1582633

[31] Cantey JB, Lee JH. Biomarkers for the diagnosis of neonatal sepsis. Clinics in Perinatology. 2021;**48**(2):215-227. DOI: 10.1016/j.clp.2021.03.012

[32] Yadav P, Yadav SK. Progress in diagnosis and treatment of neonatal sepsis: A review article. JNMA; Journal of the Nepal Medical Association. 2022;**60**(247):318-324. DOI: 10.31729/jnma.7324

[33] Sullivan BA, Hochheimer CJ, Chernyavskiy P, King WE, Fairchild KD. Impact of race on heart rate characteristics monitoring in very low birth weight infants. Pediatric Research. 2023;**94**(2):575-580. DOI: 10.1038/s41390-023-02470-z

[34] Zeigler AC, Ainsworth JE, Fairchild KD, Wynn JL, Sullivan BA. Sepsis and mortality prediction in very low birth weight infants: Analysis of HeRO and nSOFA. American Journal of Perinatology. 2023;**40**(4):407-414. DOI: 10.1055/s-0041-1728829

[35] Wynn JL, Polin RA. A neonatal sequential organ failure assessment score predicts mortality to late-onset sepsis in preterm very low birth weight infants. Pediatric Research. 2020;**88**(1):85-90. DOI: 10.1038/s41390-019-0517-2

[36] Kausch SL, Brandberg JG, Qiu J, Panda A, Binai A, Isler J, et al. Cardiorespiratory signature of neonatal sepsis: Development and validation of prediction models in 3 NICUs. Pediatric Research. 2023;**93**(7):1913-1921. DOI: 10.1038/s41390-022-02444-7. Epub 2023 Jan 2

[37] Sofouli GA, Kanellopoulou A, Vervenioti A, Dimitriou G, Gkentzi D. Predictive scores for late-onset neonatal sepsis as an early diagnostic and antimicrobial stewardship tool: What have we done so far? Antibiotics. 2022;**11**(7):928. DOI: 10.3390/antibiotics11070928

[38] Labi AK, Enweronu-Laryea CC, Nartey ET, Bjerrum S, Ayibor PK, Andersen LP, et al. Bloodstream infections at two neonatal intensive care units in Ghana: Multidrug resistant enterobacterales undermine the usefulness of standard antibiotic regimes. The Pediatric Infectious Disease Journal. 2021;**40**(12):1115-1121. DOI: 10.1097/INF.0000000000003284

[39] Lobo BBP, Marba STM, Machado HC, Caldas JPS. Neonatal

sequential organ failure assessment as a late-onset sepsis mortality predictor in very low birth weight newborns: A Brazilian cohort study. European Journal of Pediatrics. 2022;**181**(10):3767-3774. DOI: 10.1007/s00431-022-04583-9

[40] Fleiss N, Coggins SA, Lewis AN, Zeigler A, Cooksey KE, Walker LA, et al. Evaluation of the neonatal sequential organ failure assessment and mortality risk in preterm infants with late-onset infection. JAMA Network Open. 2021;**4**(2):e2036518. DOI: 10.1001/jamanetworkopen.2020.36518

[41] Barantsevich N, Barantsevich E. Diagnosis and treatment of invasive candidiasis. Antibiotics (Basel). 2022;**11**(6):718. DOI: 10.3390/antibiotics11060718

[42] Roca A, Camara B, Bognini JD, et al. Effect of intrapartum azithromycin vs placebo on neonatal sepsis and death: A randomized clinical trial. Journal of the American Medical Association. 2023;**329**(9):716-724. DOI: 10.1001/jama.2022.24388

[43] Reyman M, van Houten MA, Watson RL, et al. Effects of early-life antibiotics on the developing infant gut microbiome and resistome: A randomized trial. Nature Communications. 2022;**13**(1):893. DOI: 10.1038/s41467-022-28525-z

[44] Obiero CW, Williams P, Murunga S, et al. Randomized controlled trial of fosfomycin in neonatal sepsis: Pharmacokinetics and safety in relation to sodium overload. Archives of Disease in Childhood. 2022;**107**(9):802-810. DOI: 10.1136/archdischild-2021-322483

[45] Zhang F. Efficacy of cefotaxime combined with gamma globulins on C-reactive protein and procalcitonin in neonatal sepsis. Cellular and Molecular Biology (Noisy-le-Grand, France). 2020;**66**(2):172-176

[46] Xu YB, Ouyang Y, Zhao D. Curative effects of vancomycin and cefotaxime combined with gamma globulin respectively in neonatal septicemia and their influences on PCT, CRP and hs-CRP. European Review for Medical and Pharmacological Sciences. 2020;**24**(8):4486-4494. DOI: 10.26355/eurrev_202004_21031

[47] Reddy A, Sathenahalli V, Shivanna N, Benakappa N, Bandiya P. Ten versus 14 days of antibiotic therapy in culture-proven neonatal sepsis: A randomized, controlled trial. Indian Journal of Pediatrics. 2022;**89**(4):339-342. DOI: 10.1007/s12098-021-03794-6. Epub 2021 Jun 7

[48] Kim J, Nakwa FL, Araujo Motta F, Liu H, Dorr MB, Anderson LJ, et al. A randomized, double-blind trial investigating the efficacy of caspofungin versus amphotericin B deoxycholate in the treatment of invasive candidiasis in neonates and infants younger than 3 months of age. The Journal of Antimicrobial Chemotherapy. 2020;**75**(1):215-220. DOI: 10.1093/jac/dkz398

[49] Auriti C, Goffredo BM, Ronchetti MP, et al. High-dose micafungin in neonates and young infants with invasive candidiasis: Results of a phase 2 study. Antimicrobial Agents and Chemotherapy. Mar 2021;**65**(4):e02494-20. DOI: 10.1128/aac.02494-20

[50] Mellinghoff SC, Hoenigl M, Koehler P, Kumar A, Lagrou K, Lass-Flörl C, et al. EQUAL Candida Score: An ECMM score derived from current guidelines to measure QUAlity of Clinical Candidaemia Management. Mycoses. 2018;**61**(5):326-330. DOI: 10.1111/myc.12746

[51] Nassir KF, Al-Saddi YI, Abbas HM, et al. Pentaglobin (immunoglobulin M-enriched immunoglobulin) as adjuvant therapy for premature and very low-birth-weight neonates with sepsis. Indian Journal of Pharmacology. 2021;**53**(5):364-370. DOI: 10.4103/ijp.ijp_881_20

[52] Islam K, Khatun N, Das K, Paul S, Ghosh T, Nayek K. Ten- vs. 14-day antibiotic therapy for culture-positive neonatal sepsis. Journal of Tropical Pediatrics. 2023;**69**(6):fmad036. DOI: 10.1093/tropej/fmad036

[53] Hagag AA, El Frargy MS, Houdeeb HA. Therapeutic value of vitamin D as an adjuvant therapy in neonates with sepsis. Infectious Disorders Drug Targets. 2020;**20**(4):440-447. DOI: 10.2174/1871526519666190626141859

[54] Elfarargy MS, Al-Ashmawy G, Abu-Risha S, Khattab H. Zinc supplementation in preterm neonates with late-onset sepsis: Is it beneficial? American Journal of Perinatology. 2022;**39**(10):1097-1103. DOI: 10.1055/s-0040-1721659

[55] Kim YK, Lee J, Oh J, Rhee SJ, Shin SH, Yoon SH, et al. Population pharmacokinetic study of prophylactic fluconazole in preterm infants for prevention of invasive candidiasis. Antimicrobial Agents and Chemotherapy. 2019;**63**(6):e01960-e01918. DOI: 10.1128/AAC.01960-18

[56] Engbers AGJ, Flint RB, Voeller S, Reiss I, Liem KD, Alffenaar JC, et al. Optimization of fluconazole therapy for the treatment of invasive candidiasis in preterm infants. Archives of Disease in Childhood. 2022;**107**(4):400-406. DOI: 10.1136/archdischild-2021-322560

[57] Xie J, Zeng J, Zheng S. The efficacy and safety of fluconazole in preventing invasive fungal infection in very low birth weight infants: A systematic review and meta-analysis. Italian Journal of Pediatrics. 2023;**49**(1):51. DOI: 10.1186/s13052-023-01460-5

[58] De Rose DU, Piersigilli F, Goffredo BM, Danhaive O, Dotta A, Auriti C. Treatment with micafungin in a preterm neonate with an invasive *Candida parapsilosis* infection after a severe terlipressin-induced skin necrosis. Pathogens. 2021;**10**(7):890. DOI: 10.3390/pathogens10070890

[59] Puopolo KM, Benitz WE, Zaoutis TE, Committee on Fetus and Newborn; Committee on Infectious Diseases. Management of neonates born at ≥35 0/7 weeks' gestation with suspected or proven early-onset bacterial sepsis. Pediatrics. 2018;**142**(6):e20182894. DOI: 10.1542/peds.2018-2894

[60] Al-Lawama M, AlZaatreh A, Elrajabi R, Abdelhamid S, Badran E. Prolonged rupture of membranes, neonatal outcomes and management guidelines. Journal of Clinical Medical Research. 2019;**11**(5):360-366. DOI: 10.14740/jocmr3809

[61] Cobo T, Del Río A, Mensa J, Bosch J, Ferrero S, Palacio M. Premature rupture of membranes at term and preterm. Protocols Maternal-Fetal Medicine. 2023;**6**:1-14. Available from: https://fetalmedicinebarcelona.org/wp-content/uploads/2024/02/rotura-prematura-de-membranas-hcp-hsjd.pdf [Accessed 25 February 2025]

Chapter 2

The Role of Biomarkers in the Diagnosis of Neonatal Sepsis

Pusta Orujova, Naila Sultanova, Sevda Quliyeva, Mariam Rzayeva, Aynur Polukhova, Gulnara Mammadzada, Nushaba Panahova and Adilova Aytakin

Abstract

Neonatal sepsis remains a major cause of morbidity and mortality worldwide. Despite advances in molecular diagnostics, timely and accurate diagnosis remains a challenge, particularly in differentiating sepsis from noninfectious inflammatory conditions. Traditional microbiological culture methods are time-consuming and have limited sensitivity, leading to an increased reliance on clinical and laboratory biomarkers. This study aimed to evaluate the role of novel biomarkers, including High Mobility Group Box 1 (HMGB1), AMP-activated protein kinase (AMPK), Serum Amyloid A (sAA), and Annexin A1 (ANXA-1), in the diagnosis of neonatal sepsis. Sepsis diagnosis was based on clinical and laboratory criteria following European Medicines Agency guidelines. Routine laboratory tests and biomarker levels were assessed using SPSS statistical software. HMGB1 and AMPK levels were significantly elevated in septic neonates compared to healthy controls but lower than in neonates with non-septic infections. C-reactive protein (CRP) and PCT levels were elevated but lacked sufficient diagnostic specificity. sAA levels were lower in septic neonates but were associated with neonatal brain injury. Annexin A1 levels did not differ significantly between groups but correlated with inflammatory response markers. HMGB1 and AMPK may serve as useful biomarkers for ruling out sepsis, whereas sAA may have potential relevance in neonatal brain injury. Further large-scale studies are required to validate these findings and improve diagnostic accuracy in neonatal sepsis.

Keywords: neonatal sepsis, biomarkers, HMGB1, AMPK, annexin-1, serum amyloid A, inflammation

1. Introduction

Each year, approximately 3,000,000 newborns develop sepsis, and according to 2019 data, up to 375,000 deaths due to sepsis are recorded [1, 2]. Despite advancements in molecular diagnostics, the timely and accurate diagnosis of neonatal sepsis remains a significant challenge. Currently, the gold standard for diagnosing sepsis is a positive microbial culture. However, literature data indicate that culture-negative and suspected sepsis cases are also frequently reported.

Neonatal sepsis differs significantly from adult and pediatric sepsis, with organ dysfunction playing a more prominent role in disease progression. The Neonatal Sequential Organ Failure Assessment Score (nSOFA) is a tool used to assess neonatal organ dysfunction and serves as a potential predictor of mortality in neonatal sepsis [3]. However, even when organ dysfunction is fully evaluated, distinguishing between infection and sepsis remains difficult.

Neonatal sepsis is particularly concerning in very low birth weight infants, as it is often associated with complications due to prematurity, neurodevelopmental impairments, and increased mortality rates. These adverse outcomes underscore the importance of early sepsis recognition and prompt initiation of antibiotic therapy. However, unnecessary empirical antibiotic therapy has been linked to increased morbidity and mortality later in life, necessitating improved diagnostic and therapeutic approaches for neonatal sepsis [4–6].

Neonatal sepsis is a clinical syndrome characterized by nonspecific signs and symptoms resulting from pathogen invasion. If microbial growth is detected in blood culture or other sterile body fluids, the condition is classified as culture-positive sepsis. The existence of culture-negative sepsis and the continuation of antibiotic therapy in such cases have been long-debated issues.

Despite advancements in neonatal medicine, neonatal sepsis remains a leading cause of morbidity and mortality worldwide.

- In high-income countries, neonatal sepsis occurs in 1–4 per 1000 live births [7].
- In low- and middle-income countries, the incidence is significantly higher (49–170 per 1000 live births), with a mortality rate of up to 24%.
- Surviving infants, even those with culture-negative sepsis who receive antibiotic therapy, remain at high risk for neurodevelopmental disorders such as cerebral palsy, hearing loss, blindness, and cognitive impairments [8, 9].

The confirmed diagnosis of sepsis traditionally relies on microbiological culture techniques, which are time-consuming. Although these methods have high sensitivity for detecting low bacterial loads (1–4 CFU/mL), negative blood cultures complicate clinical assessment [10, 11].

Diagnosing culture-negative or clinical sepsis significantly increases antibiotic use (up to tenfold), inadvertently leading to necrotizing enterocolitis, fungal infections, bronchopulmonary dysplasia, and increased mortality risk. Several advancements have been made to address these challenges, including:

1. Rapid culture analysis techniques.
2. Antibiotic stewardship programs.
3. Infection prevention strategies [12].

A new molecular approach and non-culture-based methods can facilitate the timely and accurate diagnosis of sepsis. Currently, available biomarkers and additional hematologic indicators have limited value in clinical practice due to their low sensitivity and significant variability in the neonatal period, making their interpretation difficult. Ideally, the sensitivity and negative predictive value of markers should be close to 100%, while their specificity and positive predictive value should be above 85% [13]. No single marker or combination of biomarkers demonstrates adequate diagnostic accuracy for neonatal sepsis. Therefore, research is being conducted to identify new markers for diagnosing neonatal sepsis. Moreover, since infections in newborns do not always lead to sepsis, studies are also investigating factors that contribute to and increase the risk of sepsis. The main objective of this study was to examine the role of High Mobility Group Box 1 (HMGB1), AMP-activated protein kinase (AMPK), Annexin-1 (ANXA-1), and Serum Amyloid A (SAA) proteins in diagnosing neonatal sepsis. HMGB1 has been studied in the pathogenesis of various diseases, such as cancer and traumatic shock. Research has demonstrated that systemic levels of HMGB1 significantly increase in murine sepsis models, rising after 8 hours of exposure to lipopolysaccharide and reaching high levels after 16–32 hours [14, 15]. The delayed secretion of HMGB1 provides a therapeutic window for using HMGB1 antagonists in sepsis patients [16]. Studies have shown that reducing HMGB1 secretion effectively improves survival rates in septic mice [17, 18]. HMGB1 is synthesized by various immune cells, similar to proinflammatory cytokines. When these cytokines are excessively secreted, they can cause tissue damage, multiple organ dysfunction, failure, and even death. AMPK acts as a cellular stress sensor, activated through the phosphorylation of kinases in response to changes in intracellular calcium concentration or a decrease in ATP. AMPK activation reduces ATP consumption, suppresses anabolic pathways, and promotes ATP production through catabolic processes. Consequently, AMPK is a potential therapeutic target in conditions such as type 2 diabetes, cancer, and inflammatory diseases caused by energy homeostasis disturbances. AMPK activation occurs in response to pathological stresses such as glucose depletion and hypoxia. Some studies have linked AMPK activation to neurological disorders. In this context, AMPK may modulate metabolic processes during sepsis and significantly influence disease progression. Recently, the role of Serum Amyloid A (SAA) in the early diagnosis of neonatal sepsis has been investigated. This protein belongs to the lipoprotein family and is produced by the liver under the influence of cytokines [19, 20]. Some studies suggest that its synthesis occurs in the early phase of inflammation and that its diagnostic value may be higher than CRP, although different cutoff levels have been reported [21, 22]. Additionally, literature findings regarding the role of SAA in monitoring neonatal sepsis are contradictory. Therefore, investigating the diagnostic role of SAA in sepsis in comparison with clinical signs, CRP, procalcitonin, and other laboratory markers, as well as studying the association between SAA levels and the clinical course of sepsis, is of great interest.

ANXA-1, also known as lipocortin, is found in various tissues, including the lungs, kidneys, bone marrow, intestines, spleen, thymus, brain, and seminal fluid. Its extracellular activity has been extensively studied, particularly in inflammation [23, 24]. ANXA-1 must be externalized to exhibit its anti-inflammatory effects. Its release is regulated by glucocorticoids, and it inhibits phospholipase A2, thereby preventing arachidonic acid release, resulting in anti-inflammatory actions [25]. The primary anti-inflammatory effect of extracellular ANXA-1 is its ability to interfere with and modify the adhesion and migration of leukocytes, which are crucial steps in the inflammatory response [24]. ANXA-1 induces L-selectin shedding by neutrophils, likely by binding to formyl peptide receptors, leading to the detachment of adherent leukocytes from the endothelium, thus preventing their transendothelial migration [26]. The present chapter describes the results of a prospective clinical trial about the diagnostic role of proinflammatory and anti-inflammatory markers.

Material and methods: 170 newborns with 34–42 weeks' gestational age were examined. A control group consisting of 32 healthy children was formed and discharged within the first 3 days. All newborns with suspected sepsis (n = 138) were transferred to the neonatal intensive care unit (NICU) from Level I and II maternity centers in the first 2 days of life. Clinical signs of sepsis, particularly respiratory distress symptoms, were observed in all cases. In addition to an initial clinical examination, radiographic imaging of the chest and ultrasonographic evaluations of the abdomen were conducted within the first 24 hours of life. If indicated, cranial ultrasound was performed either upon admission or on the third day of life. Upon hospital admission, all newborns underwent a complete blood count (CBC) and fibrinogen, albumin, CRP, and procalcitonin assessments. Blood samples were centrifuged for biochemical analysis, and 40 microliters of plasma were separated and stored at −20°C. Plasma levels of AMPK, HMGB1, ANXA-1, and sAA proteins were measured using enzyme-linked immunosorbent assay (ELIZA) kits (Shanghai Coon Koon Biotech Co., Ltd.) following the enzyme immunoassay method. In the control group infants, the levels of AMPK, HMGB1, SAA, and ANXA-1 proteins were determined on the first day of life, while in infants admitted to the NICU with suspected sepsis, these protein levels were measured on the day of admission (either the 1st or 2nd day of life). The initial evaluation of the infants' condition was performed based on a scoring system established following the European Medicines Agency guidelines for sepsis management. The diagnosis of sepsis requires the presence of at least two clinical and two laboratory criteria. Based on these assessments, the newborns with suspected sepsis were classified into sepsis (n = 95) and non-sepsis (n = 43) (pneumonia) groups. The study then compared the analysis results between these two groups. Since sepsis symptoms appeared within the first 72 hours of life, all cases were classified as early-onset sepsis.

Statistical analysis: Statistical analysis was conducted using the SPSS 20 statistical software package on the Windows operating system. When the data showed a non-normal distribution, the Mann-Whitney test was used, while the Student's t-test was applied for normally distributed data. The Median Test, a nonparametric statistical approach and a simplified variant of the Kruskal-Wallis H test, was applied to evaluate differences in the distribution of median platelet counts between neonates with sepsis and those with pneumonia. Correlation analysis was conducted using the Pearson test for normally distributed data and the Spearman test for non-normally distributed data. To evaluate the role of the markers in diagnosing sepsis, receiver operating characteristic (ROC) analysis was performed, and sensitivity and specificity were determined.

Results: Newborns diagnosed with sepsis exhibited an increased need for mechanical ventilation. In cases of hemodynamic instability, dopamine, dobutamine, and noradrenaline infusions were administered as required. The use of fresh frozen plasma, erythrocyte mass, platelet mass, and immunological preparations was determined based on clinical indications. A detailed comparison of newborn characteristics between the two groups is presented in **Tables 1** and 2.

In the complete blood count analysis, special attention was given to the counts of white blood cells, lymphocytes, monocytes, neutrophils, and immature granulocytes on admission day. However, no statistically significant differences were found between the sepsis and non-sepsis groups (**Table 3**). Among 65 infants, procalcitonin levels showed no significant variation between the groups, whereas CRP levels were notably higher in the sepsis group. Additionally, fibrinogen levels were elevated in the sepsis group ($p < 0.001$). Lactate levels were significantly higher in the sepsis group ($p < 0.001$), whereas bicarbonate (HCO_3) and base excess (BE) levels were lower ($p < 0.001$), suggesting intensified catabolic processes and oxygen deprivation

Signs	Control Mean ± SD, Cİ lower-upper band	Sepsis Mean ± SD, Cİ lower-upper band	Non-sepsis Mean ± SD, Cİ lower-upper band	p
Pregnancy count	2.42 ± 1.39 1.91–2.93	2.46 ± 1.48 2.1–2.8	2.06 ± 1.79 1.4–2.72	* > 0.05 ** > 0.05
labor count	2.06 ± 0.93 1.72–2.4	1.96 ± 0.95 1.73–2.19	1.65 ± 0.05 1.26–2.03	* > 0.05 ** > 0.05
Age of mother	28.2 ± 5.8 25.9–30.4	28.02 ± 5.53 26.6–29.4	28.1 ± 9 24.47–31,8	* > 0.05 ** > 0.05
Gestation age	37.9 ± 1,0 37.5–38.3	36.8 ± 2 36.3–37.3	39.9 ± 1.9 36.3–37.7	* > 0.05 ** < 0.05
APGAR 1 min	7.57 ± 0.77 7.28–7.86	6.6 ± 1.34 6.18–7.01	6.64 ± 0.86 6.28–7.0	* < 0.05 ** < 0.05
APGAR 5 min	8.3 ± 0.7 8.04–8.56	7.33 ± 0.98 7.03–7.64	7.2 ± 0.71 6.91–7.49	* > 0.05 ** > 0.05
weight, gr	3098 ± 331 2977–3219	2966 ± 521 2841–3090	2904 ± 556 2841–3090	* > 0.05 ** > 0.05

*Note: SD—standard deviation, the Mann-Whitney U test, or Fisher's exact test was used, *—p comparison between control and non-sepsis group, **—p comparison between control and sepsis group.*

Table 1.
Group characteristic.

Parameters		Control	Sepsis	Non-sepsis	Pearson Chi-square
Gestation age	34–36 weeks	2 (6.5%)	20 (31.7%)	10 (34.5%)	$\chi^2 = 8.3$ p = 0.016
	37–42 weeks	29 (93.5%)	43 (68.3%)	19 (65.5%)	
Sex	girls	13 (41.9%)	29 (45.3%)	14 (46.7%)	$\chi^2 = 0.152$ p = 0.927
	boys	18 (58.1%)	35 (54.7%)	16 (53.3%)	
Type of delivery	vaginal delivery	5 (15.5%)	51 (53.7%)	23 (53.5%)	$\chi^2 = 15.07$ p = 0.001
	cesarean section	27 (84.4%)	44 (46.3%)	20 (46.5%)	
Mechanical ventilation		0	26 (28.3%)	1 (2.3%)	$\chi^2 = 22.18$ p = 0.001
Inotropic support (dopamine infusion)		0	22 (23.9%)	0	$\chi^2 = 20.65$ p = 0.001
Mortality		0	15 (16%)	0	$\chi^2 = 13.3$ p = 0.001

Table 2.
Frequency distribution of GA, sex, type of delivery, mechanical ventilation, inotropic support, and mortality across groups.

due to infection. Vital sign fluctuations are common in sepsis and require continuous monitoring for effective disease management. Although there was no statistically significant difference in platelet counts (p > 0.05), however, in the sepsis group, the majority of neonates had platelet counts below 150,000. (p = 0.024).

Indicators	Groups	N	Mean	Std. Deviation	Std. Error	95% Confidence Interval for Mean		Minimum	Maximum	median	IQR	P
						Lower Bound	Upper Bound					
PCT	sepsis	51	12.38	17.56	2.46	7.44	17.32	.06	87.40	4.76	11.07	
	non-sepsis	14	4.95	6.27	1.67	1.33	8.57	.08	18.71	1.76	6.96	.130
WBC	sepsis	86	17.88	22.55	2.39	13.13	22.62	2.38	142.00	13.5	7.42	
	non-sepsis	42	14.53	5.14	0.79	12.93	16.14	5.91	25.40	14.4	8.95	.367
PLT	sepsis	86	238.31	101.26	10.79	216.86	259.77	11.00	516.00	249	123	
	non-sepsis	42	284.02	126.53	19.52	244.59	323.45	66.00	788.00	274.5	124	.053
Neutrophil	sepsis	74	8.78	6.98	0.81	7.16	10.39	.31	51.26	8.1	6.47	
	non-sepsis	42	8.69	4.27	0.66	7.36	10.02	1.42	18.73	8.9	6.05	.452
monocyte	Sepsis	75	1.73	2.82	0.33	1.08	2.38	.04	25.00	1.44	1	
	non-sepsis	42	2.18	2.19	0.34	1.50	2.86	.54	10.60	1.6	1.1	.073
lymphocyte	sepsis	75	4.08	3.33	0.38	3.32	4.85	.38	23.83	3.4	2.6	
	non-sepsis	42	3.83	2.06	0.32	3.18	4.47	.60	11.50	3.7	2.6	.759
Ig	sepsis	73	0.41	1.48	0.17	0.07	0.76	.01	12.63	0.14	0.3	
	non-sepsis	41	0.26	0.38	0.06	0.14	0.38	.01	1.87	0.14	0.22	.793
Neu/lym	sepsis	75	4.02	3.40	0.40	3.22	4.82	.08	23.83	2.4	2.38	
	non-sepsis	42	3.83	2.06	0.32	3.18	4.47	.60	11.50	2.5	3.1	.622
Ig/leucocyte	sepsis	69	1.75	2.17	0.26	1.23	2.27	.06	13.76	0.01	0.015	
	non-sepsis	41	1.55	2.04	0.32	0.91	2.20	.14	10.73	0.008	0.02	.257
Plt/ lymphocyte	sepsis	74	92.38	82.01	9.53	73.38	111.38	4.49	453.57	71.8	60	
	non-sepsis	42	98.86	75.71	11.68	75.27	122.45	12.67	371.67	80.6	68.7	.567

Indicators	Groups	N	Mean	Std. Deviation	Std. Error	95% Confidence Interval for Mean		Minimum	Maximum	median	IQR	p
						Lower Bound	Upper Bound					
C-reactive protein	sepsis	88	33.56	50.30	5.36	22.91	44.22	.11	258.50	11.6	45.7	
	non-sepsis	38	9.05	15.27	2.48	4.03	14.07	.02	66.00	1.8	7.3	.000
Albumin	sepsis	45	9.18	11.44	1.71	5.74	12.62	1.60	36.76	2.5	0.5	
	non-sepsis	7	9.37	11.41	4.31	−1.18	19.92	2.20	30.44	2.9	1	.259
ALT	sepsis	31	46.03	110.58	19.86	5.47	86.59	2.46	626.00	14.4	28.6	
	non-sepsis	9	12.46	3.96	1.32	9.42	15.51	7.00	20.00	11	5.42	.270
ACT	sepsis	31	86.93	158.38	28.45	28.84	145.03	17.00	888.00	41.5	34	
	non-sepsis	9	35.23	20.56	6.85	19.42	51.04	17.00	83.00	31	25	.056
Fibrinogen	sepsis	60	223.73	90.08	11.63	200.46	247.00	96.00	501.00	203	118	
	non-sepsis	28	191.50	101.11	19.11	152.29	230.71	92.00	514.00	153	96	.030
lactate	sepsis	73	3.18	2.25	0.26	2.65	3.70	.80	11.80	2.5	1.6	
	non-sepsis	22	1.77	0.87	0.19	1.38	2.16	.70	5.00	1.5	0.74	.000
HCO3	sepsis	72	20.20	4.37	0.52	19.17	21.23	4.80	32.40	20.7	3.6	
	non-sepsis	22	22.18	3.26	0.70	20.73	23.62	17.30	30.00	21.4	5.4	.038
BE	sepsis	72	−5.16	4.29	0.51	−6.16	−4.15	−24.00	8.10	−4.5	4.5	
	non-sepsis	23	−3.08	3.27	0.68	−4.50	−1.67	−9.90	3.20	−3	4.3	.021

Note: PCT—procalcitonin (ng/ml), WBC—white blood cell (10^3/μL), PLT-platelet (*10^3/μL), neutrophil (*10^3/μL), monocyte (*10^3/μL), lymphocyte (*10^3/μL), Ig-immature granulocytes (*10^3/μL), Neu/lym-neutrophil Lymphocyte ratio, Ig/leu-immature granulocyte leucocyte ratio, Plt/lym-platelet lymphocyte ratio, ALT-alanine aminotransferase (U/L), ACT-aspartate aminotransferase (U/L), Fibrinogen (mg/dL), lactate (mmol/L), HCO3-Bicarbonate (mmol/L), BE-Base excess (mmol/L).*

Table 3.
Comparison levels of blood cell counts, the calculated value of Neu/lym, Plt/lym, IG\WBC, ALT, ACT, Fibrinogen, Albumin, lactate, HCO3, BE, procalcitonin and CRP levels.

Levels of AMPK and HMGB1 were higher in the sepsis group compared to the control group infants but lower than the non-sepsis group infants (AMPK median level in the control group, 934.4 pg./ml; in sepsis group, 1093 pg./ml; in pneumonia group, 1420 pg./ml; among all groups, $p = 0.001$). Similarly, HMGB1 levels followed the same pattern as AMPK, being higher in septic infants than in healthy ones but lower than in infants with pneumonia (median levels in: control—1037 pg./ml, sepsis—1484 pg./ml, non-septic—1643 pg./ml) (**Figure 1**). When the median test was performed, 24 out of 57 septic infants had HMGB1 levels above the median, whereas 19 out of 29 in the non-septic group had levels above the median ($p < 0.05$). Among infants who died, HMGB1 levels were higher compared to survivors, but the difference was not statistically significant ($p > 0.05$). Conversely, AMPK levels were lower in deceased infants ($p > 0.05$). When analyzing the correlation between markers, a direct correlation was found between hospital stay and procalcitonin (PCT) levels ($r = 0.320$, $p = 0.022$), while an inverse correlation was observed with AMPK levels ($r = -0.226$, $p = 0.028$). Additionally, a direct correlation was found between AMPK and HMGB1 levels ($r = 0.336$, $p = 0.001$). However, in deceased infants, a negative correlation was noted between AMPK and HMGB1 levels ($r = -0.524$; $p > 0.05$) (**Figure 2**).

The sAA median levels were 4.1 mcg/ml in the control group, 3.6 mcg/ml in the sepsis group, and 4.0 mcg/ml in the pneumonia group. The median sAA level in the sepsis group was lower compared to both other groups, and this difference was statistically significant ($p_{0-1} < 0.05$; $p_{1-2} < 0.05$). For ANXA-1, the median level was 11.1 pg./ml in the control group, 10.5 pg./ml in the sepsis group, and 11.0 pg./ml in the pneumonia and infection group, with no statistically significant difference between the groups. Given that ANXA-1 plays a role in maintaining blood-brain barrier permeability, its levels were also examined in septic infants with suspected brain injuries. In these cases, a slight decrease in ANXA-1 levels was noted. 134 underwent cranial ultrasound, and brain injuries were detected in 57 infants. In the sepsis group, neurosonography revealed changes in 37 children, including intraventricular hemorrhage (grade 1 in 17 children, grade 2 in 12 children, and grade 3 in 2 children), ventriculitis in one child, ischemic foci in one child, increased echogenicity of the periventricular area in one child, and cerebral edema in one child. In the pneumonia group, changes were noted in 20 children, including intraventricular hemorrhage (grade 1 in 8 children and grade 2 in 5 children), vasculopathy in one child, ischemic foci in the brain tissue in five children, and periventricular edema in one child ($p = 0.004$). The median level of ANXA-1 was 11.7 pg./ml in children with documented brain injuries and 11.6 pg./ml in children without detected injuries ($p > 0.05$). However, ANXA-1 levels did not provide informative value for infants with brain injuries. On the other hand, sAA protein, as an inflammatory marker, was lower in septic infants but showed diagnostic significance in cases with brain injuries. The mean sAA level was 4.1 ± 1 mcg/ml in infants with brain injuries, compared to 3.4 ± 1 mcg/ml in those without ($p < 0.05$). Although ANXA-1 did not reach statistical significance, a direct correlation was found between ANXA-1 and sAA ($r = 0.338$, $p = 0.029$), suggesting that ANXA-1 may increase during inflammatory processes and play a protective role. According to the ROC analysis, among the studied proteins, only AMPK and HMGB1 were significant for ruling out sepsis at the first suspicion of infection. To rule out sepsis, the cutoff level for AMPK was 971, with a sensitivity of 57% and a specificity of 32%, while the cutoff level for HMGB1 was 1436.5, with a sensitivity of 54% and a specificity of 36%. However, commonly used routine markers such as CRP and PCT were not statistically significant for confirming the diagnosis of sepsis (**Figure 3**).

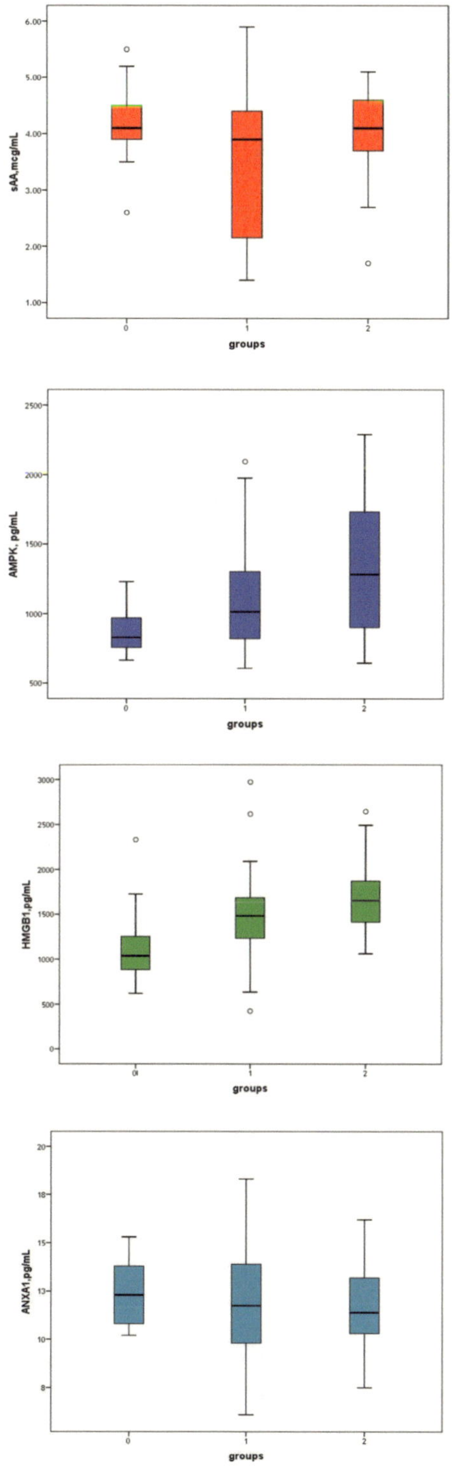

Figure 1.
AMPK, HMGB1, ANXA-1, and sAA protein levels in groups. Note: Groups: 0—control; 1—sepsis; 2—pneumonia and infection. AMPK $p_{0-1} < 0.05$; $p_{0-2} < 0.05$; $p_{1-2} < 0.05$; *HMGB-1* $p_{0-1} < 0.05$; $p_{0-2} < 0.05$; $p_{1-2} < 0.05$; *ANXA; 1* $p_{0-1} > 0.05$; $p_{0-2} > 0.05$; $p_{1-2} > 0.05$; *sAA* $p_{0-1} < 0.05$; $p_{0-2} > 0.05$; $p_{1-2} = 0.05$.

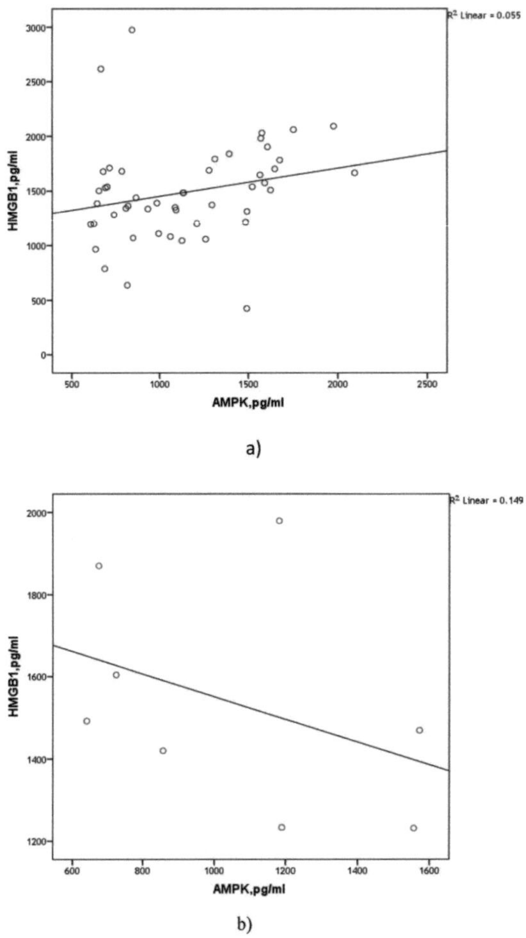

Figure 2.
Correlation between AMPK and HMGB-1 (a) in survived septic babies (b) in deceased septic babies.

2. Discussion

The early diagnosis of neonatal sepsis continues to pose significant clinical and diagnostic challenges due to its subtle and nonspecific clinical manifestations, the delayed nature of culture results, and the low sensitivity of traditional laboratory parameters.

In this context, the present study contributes valuable insights into the utility of novel biomarkers—HMGB1, AMPK, sAA, and ANXA-1—for improving diagnostic accuracy and risk stratification in neonatal sepsis. The role of inflammatory markers in the early diagnosis of neonatal sepsis remains a subject of ongoing debate. While some studies have demonstrated the superior diagnostic value of PCT, others highlight the higher informativeness of CRP. In our study, CRP levels were found to rise earlier than PCT levels in confirming the clinical diagnosis of sepsis. Specifically, we observed elevated CRP concentrations as early as the first or second day of life, coinciding with the infants' admission to the NICU. Previous research has also emphasized the prognostic value of fibrinogen in pediatric populations, with levels below 2 g/L being associated with increased mortality risk [27]. Our findings align

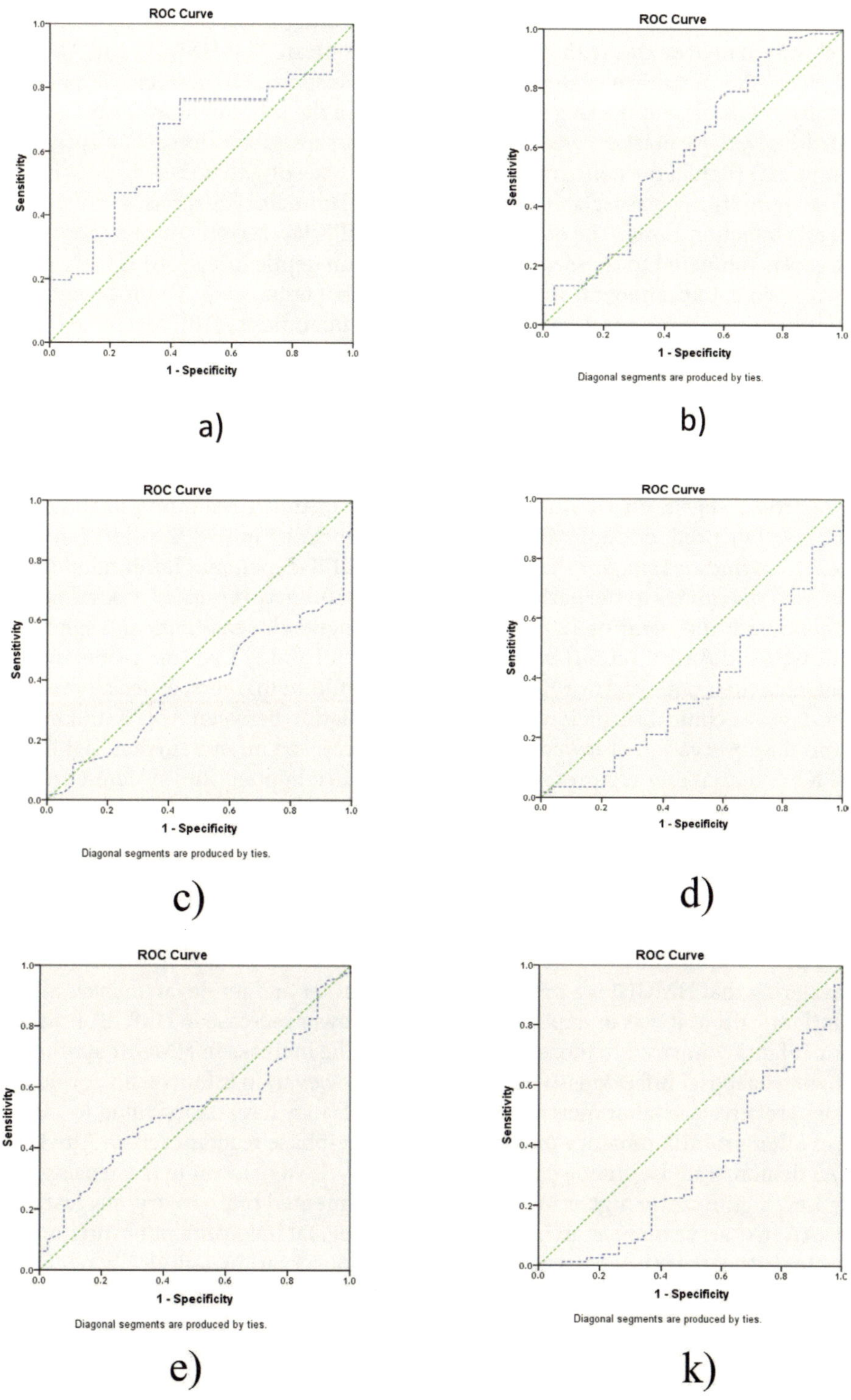

Figure 3.
ROC analysis of proteins level in neonates with suspected sepsis for diagnosis of sepsis. (a) PCT; AUC = 0.633,p > 0.05; (b) CRP 1st day; AUC = 0.590. p > 0.05; (c)sAA-AUC = 0.386. p > 0.05; (d) HMGB-1; AUC = 0.362. p < 0.05; (e) AMPK; AUC = 0.332. p < 0.05; (k) ANXA-1; AUC = 0.528. p > 0.05.

with these observations, reinforcing the diagnostic and prognostic utility of fibrinogen elevation in neonates with sepsis. Our results indicate that HMGB1 and AMPK levels were significantly elevated in neonates with suspected infections compared to healthy controls, supporting their involvement in the inflammatory response. Interestingly, these markers were higher in the non-sepsis infection group (primarily pneumonia) than in the confirmed sepsis group, suggesting that their expression may be more strongly associated with localized inflammatory responses rather than systemic infection alone. The observation that AMPK levels were lower in neonates with sepsis compared to those with pneumonia (non-septic infection) is biologically plausible. Experimental studies have shown that enhancing AMPK activity accelerates the recovery of damaged lung tissue in pneumonia [28]. Mechanistically, AMPK deficiency leads to increased PKM2-dependent aerobic glycolysis, resulting in enhanced release of HMGB1—a late-phase proinflammatory mediator—from macrophages and monocytes. Accordingly, pharmacological activation of AMPK (e.g., with A-769662) has been shown to confer protection, while depletion of AMPKα in myeloid cells exacerbates outcomes in murine models of endotoxic shock and polymicrobial sepsis. Furthermore, administration of the PKM2 inhibitor shikonin reduces lactate production, HMGB1 release, and mortality in AMPKα-deficient mice. These findings suggest that disruption of AMPK-dependent immunometabolic pathways contributes to the pathogenesis of sepsis and may represent a novel target for therapeutic intervention [29]. The moderate diagnostic sensitivity and specificity of HMGB1 and AMPK (cutoff values of 1436.5 pg./ml and 971 pg./ml, respectively) underscore their potential as rule-out rather than rule-in markers, especially in the early stages of clinical suspicion. The inverse correlation between AMPK and mortality and the observation of lower AMPK levels in deceased infants further highlight AMPK's potential role as a protective mediator against hypoxia and systemic stress. Since AMPK plays a protective role against hypoxia by increasing ATP consumption during inflammation, the presence of this inverse correlation in deceased infants highlights the significance of AMPK in the disease process. This finding aligns with previous studies suggesting that AMPK activation facilitates energy homeostasis and may attenuate cellular damage during inflammatory stress. The inverse correlation between AMPK and hospital stay also supports its potential as a prognostic marker. Considering that HMGB1 is a proinflammatory marker and its elevated levels accelerate inflammation, it was unexpected to observe a lower increase in HMGB1 levels in septic infants compared to those with infections. The increase in HMGB1 synthesis following bacterial infection is well understood. However, in infants who developed sepsis, a relatively smaller increase in HMGB1 levels may have contributed to a lower rise in other proinflammatory mediators. The acute-phase reactant serum Amyloid A (sAA) demonstrated a unique pattern: although levels were lower in the sepsis group, they were significantly higher in infants with documented brain injury, suggesting that sAA may serve more as an indicator of neurological involvement or inflammatory neurotoxicity rather than systemic infection. This observation is clinically relevant, as early identification of neurological complications in septic neonates remains a major unmet need in neonatal intensive care. The role of ANXA-1 was less conclusive in this study. Although ANXA-1 did not differ significantly across groups, its positive correlation with sAA and trend toward lower levels in infants with brain injury suggest a possible anti-inflammatory or neuroprotective role, consistent with its known function in maintaining blood-brain barrier integrity. However, the lack of statistical significance limits its standalone diagnostic utility, and its relevance may be better understood as part of a biomarker panel. Routine inflammatory markers such as CRP and PCT demonstrated limited diagnostic value in this cohort, reinforcing the need for more specific and early-detecting markers. Notably, PCT correlated significantly with the need for inotropic support, aligning with its known association with disease severity rather than initial diagnosis. The analysis of metabolic parameters revealed significantly higher lactate and lower bicarbonate and base excess in septic neonates, indicating a shift toward anaerobic metabolism and systemic hypoperfusion. These parameters remain critical adjuncts to clinical and biomarker evaluation, particularly in hemodynamically unstable infants. Despite these findings, the study has several limitations. The relatively modest sample size and the inclusion of a diverse clinical spectrum under the non-sepsis group may have influenced biomarker distribution and statistical power. Lastly, while this study sheds light on biomarker behavior at early clinical suspicion, the lack of culture-positive confirmation in many cases mirrors real-world challenges but also complicates definitive validation of diagnostic performance.

3. Conclusion

Neonatal sepsis remains a major diagnostic and clinical challenge due to its nonspecific presentation, the limitations of traditional microbiological culture techniques, and the need for timely and accurate identification. Biomarkers play an essential role in enhancing the diagnostic process, particularly when culture results are inconclusive or delayed. In this study, HMGB1 and AMPK were identified as potential biomarkers for ruling out sepsis, while sAA showed relevance in cases with neonatal brain injury. ANXA-1, although not statistically significant across different groups, demonstrated a correlation with inflammatory markers, suggesting a possible protective role in inflammation-related processes. Despite advances in biomarker research, no single marker or combination of biomarkers currently provides adequate diagnostic accuracy for neonatal sepsis. Further large-scale studies are necessary to validate these findings and refine biomarker-based diagnostic strategies. The integration of novel molecular techniques, along with improved clinical assessment tools, may lead to enhanced diagnostic precision, more targeted therapeutic approaches, and ultimately better neonatal outcomes.

Conflict of interest

The authors declare no conflict of interest.

Notes

The study was approved by the Ethics Committee of Azerbaijan Medical University on December 8, 2023 (Protocol No. 29).

Thanks

We extend our deepest gratitude to the leadership and staff of the Scientific Research Institute of Pediatrics named after Kubra Farajova, the Scientific Research

Institute of Obstetrics and Gynecology, and the Republican Perinatal Center of the Ministry of Health of the Republic of Azerbaijan for facilitating the collection of research materials. We also sincerely thank the leadership and staff of the Scientific Research Center of Azerbaijan Medical University for their assistance in conducting laboratory examinations.

Author details

Pusta Orujova[1*], Naila Sultanova[2], Sevda Quliyeva[3], Mariam Rzayeva[4], Aynur Polukhova[5], Gulnara Mammadzada[6], Nushaba Panahova[7] and Adilova Aytakin[7]

1 2nd Child Disease Department Azerbaijan Medical University, Baku, Azerbaijan

2 II Department of Children's Diseases, Azerbaijan Medical University, Azerbaijan

3 Scientific Research Center, Azerbaijan Medical University, Azerbaijan

4 Azerbaijan Republic Perinatal Center, Azerbaijan

5 Scientific Research Institute of Pediatrics Named after Kubra Faradjova, Azerbaijan

6 Scientific Research Institute of Gynaecology and Obstetrics, Azerbaijan

7 Scientific Research Institute of Paediatrics Named after Kubra Faradjova, Baku, Azerbaijan

*Address all correspondence to: pusteeli@gmail.com

References

[1] Fleischmann-Struzek C et al. The global burden of paediatric and neonatal sepsis: A systematic review. The Lancet Respiratory Medicine. 2018;**6**:223-230

[2] United Nations Inter-agency Group for Child Mortality Estimation (UN IGME). Levels and Trends in Child Mortality: Report. Estimates Developed by the United Nations Inter-Agency Group for Child Mortality Estimation. New York: United Nations Children's Fund; 2019. p. 2019

[3] Wynn J, Polin RA. A neonatal sequential organ failure assessment score predicts mortality to late-onset sepsis in preterm very low birth weight infants. Pediatric Research. 2020;**88**:85-90

[4] Liu L, Johnson HL, Cousens S, Perin J, Scott S, Lawn JE, et al. Global, regional, and national causes of child mortality: An updated systematic analysis for 2010 with time trends since 2000. Lancet. 2012;**379**:2151-2161. DOI: 10.1016/S0140-6736(12)60560-1

[5] WHO. Newborns: Improving Survival and Well-Being. Geneva: World Health Organisation; 2020

[6] Chiesa C, Panero A, Osborn JF, Simonetti AF, Pacifico L. Diagnosis of neonatal sepsis: A clinical and laboratory challenge. Clinical Chemistry. 2004;**50**:279-287. DOI: 10.1373/clinchem.2003.025171

[7] Fleischmann-Struzek C, Goldfarb DM, Schlattmann P, Schlapbach LJ, Reinhart K, Kissoon N. The global burden of paediatric and neonatal sepsis: A systematic review. The Lancet Respiratory Medicine. 2018;**6**:223-230. DOI: 10.1016/S2213-2600(18)30063-8

[8] Li Y, Ji M, Yang J. Current understanding of long-term cognitive impairment after sepsis. Frontiers in Immunology. 2022;**13**:855006. DOI: 10.3389/fimmu.2022.855006

[9] Alshaikh B, Yusuf K, Sauve R. Neurodevelopmental outcomes of very low birth weight infants with neonatal sepsis: Systematic review and meta-analysis. Journal of Perinatology. 2013;**33**:558-564. DOI: 10.1038/jp.2012.167

[10] Jardine L, Davies MW, Faoagali J. Incubation time required for neonatal blood cultures to become positive. Journal of Paediatrics and Child Health. 2006;**42**:797-802. DOI: 10.1111/j.1440-1754.2006.00980.x

[11] Sarkar S, Bhagat I, DeCristofaro JD, Wiswell TE, Spitzer AR. A study of the role of multiple site blood cultures in the evaluation of neonatal sepsis. Journal of Perinatology. 2006;**26**:18-22. DOI: 10.1038/sj.jp.7211410

[12] CDC. Core Elements of Antibiotic Stewardship. 2021e. Available from: https://www.cdc.gov/antibiotic-use/core-elements/index.html

[13] Monaghan TF et al. Foundational statistical principles in medical research: Sensitivity, specificity, positive predictive value, and negative predictive value. Medicina (Kaunas, Lithuania). 2021;**57**(5):503. DOI: 10.3390/medicina57050503

[14] Venereau E, De Leo F, Mezzapelle R, Careccia G, Musco G, Bianchi ME. HMGB1 as biomarker and drug target. Pharmacological Research. 2016;**111**:534-544. DOI: 10.1016/j.phrs.2016.06.031

[15] Yu Y, Tang D, Kang R. Oxidative stress-mediated HMGB1 biology. Frontiers in Physiology. 2015;**6**:93. DOI: 10.3389/fphys.2015.00093

[16] Deng M, Tang Y, Li W, Wang X, Zhang R, Zhang X, et al. The endotoxin delivery protein HMGB1 mediates caspase-11-dependent lethality in sepsis. Immunity. 2018;**49**:740-53. e7. DOI: 10.1016/j.immuni.2018.08.016

[17] Yang H, Wang H, Chavan SS, Andersson U. High mobility group box protein 1 (HMGB1): The prototypical endogenous danger molecule. Molecular Medicine. 2015;**21**(Suppl 1):S6-S12. DOI: 10.2119/molmed.2015.00087

[18] Yang S, Lee W, Lee BS, Lee C, Park EK, Ku SK, et al. Aloin reduces HMGB1-mediated septic responses and improves survival in septic mice by activation of the SIRT1 and PI3K/Nrf2/HO-1 signaling Axis. The American Journal of Chinese Medicine. 2019;**47**:613-633. DOI: 10.1142/S0192415X19500320

[19] Carling D, Sanders MJ, Woods A. The regulation of AMP-activated protein kinase by upstream kinases. International Journal of Obesity. 2008;**32**(Suppl 4):S55-S59. DOI: 10.1038/ijo.2008.124

[20] Steinberg GR, Kemp BE. AMPK in health and disease. Physiological Reviews. 2009;**89**:1025-1078. DOI: 10.1152/physrev.00011.2008

[21] Yuan H, Huang J, Lv B, Yan W, Hu G, Wang J, et al. Diagnosis value of the serum amyloid A test in neonatal sepsis: A meta-analysis. BioMed Research International. 2013;**2013**:520294. DOI: 10.1155/2013/520294. Epub 2013 Aug 5

[22] Dorum BA, Özkan H, Çakir SÇ, Köksal N, GÖZAL Z, Çelebi S, et al. The diagnostic value of serum amyloid a in early-onset neonatal sepsis in premature infants. The Journal of Pediatrics. 2021;**26**:8-13

[23] Xu R, Weber MC, Hu X, Neumann PA, Kamaly N. Annexin A1 based inflammation resolving mediators and nanomedicines for inflammatory bowel disease therapy. Seminars in Immunology. 2022;**61-64**:101664. DOI: 10.1016/j.smim.2022.101664

[24] Kelly L, McGrath S, Rodgers L, et al. Annexin-A1: The culprit or the solution? Immunology. 2022;**166**:2-16. DOI: 10.1111/imm.13455

[25] Liu H, He J, Wu Y, et al. Endothelial regulation by exogenous annexin A1 in inflammatory response and BBB integrity following traumatic brain injury. Frontiers in Neuroscience. 2021;**15**:627110. DOI: 10.3389/fnins.2021.627110

[26] Bruschi M, Petretto A, Vaglio A, Santucci L, Candiano G, Ghiggeri GM. Annexin A1 and autoimmunity: From basic science to clinical applications. International Journal of Molecular Sciences. 2018;**19**:1348. DOI: 10.3390/ijms19051348

[27] Shao XTL et al. Fibrinogen as a prognostic predictor in pediatric patients with sepsis: A database study. Mediators of Inflammation. 2020;**2020**:9153620. DOI: 10.1155/2020/9153620

[28] Jr EB, Husain M, Bone N, Smith S, Morris P, Zmijewski JW. AMPK activation improves recovery from pneumonia-induced lung injury via reduction of er-stress and apoptosis in alveolar epithelial cells. Respiratory Research. 2023;**24**:185. DOI: 10.1186/s12931-023-02483-6

[29] Huang J, Liu K, et al. AMPK regulates immunometabolism in sepsis. Brain, Behaviour, and Immunity. 2018;**72**:89-100

Chapter 3

Perspective Chapter: Parenteral Nutrition in NICU

Hossam A. Elgnainy

Abstract

Parenteral nutrition is a vital therapeutic intervention in neonatal intensive care units for neonates unable to receive adequate nutrition through enteral feeding. It is especially essential for preterm or critically ill infants with immature gastrointestinal systems. Parenteral nutrition provides necessary nutrients, including carbohydrates, proteins, fats, vitamins, and minerals, directly into the bloodstream, bypassing the gastrointestinal tract. This intervention supports growth, metabolic balance, and overall health outcomes. Neonates with medical conditions such as gastrointestinal malformations, prematurity, or respiratory distress syndrome often rely on parenteral nutrition for survival and development. Parenteral nutrition is critical in preventing malnutrition, growth failure, and related complications. In particular, preterm infants with underdeveloped organ systems require customized nutritional support, which parenteral nutrition facilitates. Parenteral nutrition is crucial for critically ill neonates, providing essential nutrients for immune function, tissue repair, and recovery. Parenteral nutrition plays a significant role in improving developmental outcomes and long-term health.

Keywords: parenteral nutrition, neonatal intensive care unit, preterm infants, critical care, gastrointestinal system, nutritional support, malnutrition, growth failure, immune function, neurodevelopmental outcomes

1. Introduction

Parenteral nutrition (PN) is a critical therapeutic intervention used in the neonatal intensive care unit (NICU) to provide essential nutrients to neonates who cannot receive adequate nutrition through enteral feeding. Neonates, particularly those who are preterm or critically ill, often have immature or compromised gastrointestinal systems, making it challenging to meet their nutritional requirements via oral or enteral feeds. PN becomes an essential tool for ensuring that these vulnerable infants receive the nutrients necessary for growth and development.

Parenteral nutrition involves the intravenous administration of a specially formulated solution containing carbohydrates, proteins, fats, vitamins, minerals, and electrolytes. This method of nutritional support is essential for maintaining metabolic balance, promoting growth, and preventing nutrient deficiencies that can impact development and overall health outcomes.

The use of PN in neonates requires careful consideration, as the neonatal period is a time of rapid growth and development. The nutritional needs of neonates are highly specific, and achieving the right balance of nutrients is crucial for their survival and long-term health [1].

1.1 The role of parenteral nutrition in neonatal intensive care

In the NICU, neonates may face a variety of medical conditions that prevent them from being able to consume adequate nutrition orally. Conditions such as gastrointestinal malformations, prematurity, respiratory distress syndrome, or severe infections can disrupt the neonate's ability to take in and process nutrition through the gastrointestinal tract. In such cases, PN provides a lifeline, ensuring that essential nutrients are delivered directly into the bloodstream to sustain vital functions and promote growth.

PN is often used when the digestive system is immature or when the neonate requires time to stabilize before being introduced to enteral feeds. The provision of parenteral nutrition in these cases helps reduce the risk of malnutrition, growth failure, and related complications [2].

1.2 Understanding parenteral nutrition

Parenteral nutrition is particularly critical for preterm infants, as their nutritional needs are often more complex and urgent due to their underdeveloped organ systems. Preterm neonates are prone to issues such as inadequate gut motility, enzyme deficiencies, and a higher risk of infection. PN allows clinicians to provide customized nutritional support based on the individual needs of each neonate, adjusting the formulation as necessary to address their changing condition and growth requirements.

By delivering nutrients intravenously, PN bypasses the gastrointestinal tract, providing neonates with the necessary nutrients without placing additional stress on their immature systems. This approach is vital in supporting neonates through the critical early stages of life, setting the foundation for healthy growth and development [3].

2. Importance of parenteral nutrition in neonatal care

Parenteral nutrition (PN) plays a crucial role in the care of neonates, particularly those who are premature, critically ill, or suffering from conditions that impair their ability to ingest or absorb nutrition through normal feeding routes. The neonatal period, marked by rapid growth and development, places significant demands on the body's nutritional needs, and PN becomes an essential therapeutic tool when the gastrointestinal system is unable to meet these needs.

Neonates, especially preterm infants, face various challenges that may hinder their ability to take in or process enteral nutrition. These challenges include immaturity of the gastrointestinal tract, poor gut motility, and increased vulnerability to gastrointestinal complications like necrotizing enterocolitis (NEC). Parenteral nutrition ensures that these neonates receive the essential nutrients required for survival, development, and optimal growth, especially in the early stages of life when nutrient demands are highest [3].

2.1 Essential nutritional support for critically ill neonates

Critically ill neonates are often presented with complex medical conditions such as congenital malformations, respiratory distress syndrome (RDS), or infections. In these cases, the infant's ability to tolerate oral or enteral feeding can be severely limited, and PN offers an alternative method of delivering nutrition that bypasses the gastrointestinal tract entirely. This allows for direct nutrient absorption into the bloodstream, supporting vital functions such as cellular growth, immune function, and tissue repair.

By providing an adequate supply of nutrients during this critical period, PN helps reduce the risk of complications such as malnutrition, which can impair immune function, growth, and development. It also supports the neonate's ability to recover from illness or surgery, ensuring that the infant's body has the necessary resources to fight infections, heal wounds, and build healthy tissues [1].

2.2 Parenteral nutrition as a cornerstone of neonatal critical care

In the NICU, where neonates are closely monitored and managed for a wide range of health issues, PN serves as a cornerstone of neonatal care. It is not only a lifesaving intervention for critically ill infants but also a cornerstone of recovery and growth. PN allows neonates to receive all the necessary macronutrients (carbohydrates, proteins, and lipids) and micronutrients (vitamins, minerals, and trace elements) essential for development, even when they cannot consume or digest food orally [2, 4].

2.3 A lifesaving tool for preterm and low birth weight infants

For preterm infants, particularly those born with very low birth weight (VLBW) or extremely low birth weight (ELBW), PN is often the only means of achieving sufficient nutrition in the early days of life. These infants may require weeks or even months of nutritional support through PN until they reach the stage where they can tolerate enteral feeding. Providing adequate PN ensures that they do not suffer from malnutrition or growth failure, both of which can have long-term consequences for their health.

In addition to meeting basic nutritional needs, PN in neonates can prevent the harmful effects of nutrient deficiencies, such as delayed brain development, weakened immune response, and poor wound healing. Ensuring proper nutrient provision in the neonatal period can have lasting positive effects on neurodevelopmental outcomes and overall health [5].

3. Indications for parenteral nutrition in the NICU

Parenteral nutrition (PN) is a vital intervention for neonates who are unable to receive adequate nutrition *via* oral or enteral feeding. In the neonatal intensive care unit (NICU), several clinical conditions and factors may necessitate the use of PN to ensure the neonate's nutritional needs are met, thereby supporting growth, metabolic stability, and recovery [6].

3.1 Identifying neonates who require parenteral nutrition

The decision to initiate PN is based on a neonate's ability to absorb and process nutrients *via* the gastrointestinal tract. When enteral feeding is contraindicated or insufficient, PN becomes the primary alternative for delivering the necessary nutrients. The following are common indications for PN in the NICU [2, 7]:

1. *Prematurity and low birth weight*: Premature infants, especially those with very low birth weight (VLBW) or extremely low birth weight (ELBW), often experience significant difficulties with enteral feeding due to their underdeveloped gastrointestinal systems. These infants are frequently unable to meet their nutritional requirements through oral or enteral feeds, and PN is crucial for providing the nutrients necessary to promote growth and development during the early stages of life [3].

2. *Gastrointestinal malformations or surgical interventions*: Neonates with congenital gastrointestinal anomalies such as gastroschisis, omphalocele, or intestinal atresia may require PN for extended periods, particularly following surgical interventions. These conditions can prevent normal feeding, and PN becomes essential for providing the neonate with vital nutrients while the gastrointestinal tract heals or matures [8].

3. *Necrotizing enterocolitis (NEC)*: Necrotizing enterocolitis (NEC) is a life-threatening gastrointestinal condition that affects preterm and low birth weight infants. In cases where NEC leads to bowel perforation or extensive bowel damage, enteral feeding is often contraindicated. PN provides a safe and effective means of nutritional support during the acute phase of the disease and while the infant's gastrointestinal system recovers [9].

4. *Inability to tolerate enteral feeds*: Some neonates may experience feeding intolerance, characterized by symptoms such as vomiting, abdominal distension, or delayed gastric emptying. These issues can occur due to immaturity of the digestive system or underlying conditions like gastrointestinal reflux or metabolic disorders. PN is often required in such cases to ensure the infant receives adequate nutrition while their digestive system stabilizes or matures [10].

5. *Severe respiratory or cardiovascular illness*: Neonates with severe respiratory distress syndrome (RDS), congenital heart defects, or other serious conditions affecting oxygenation or circulation may be unable to tolerate enteral feeding. In these cases, PN is indicated to ensure the neonate's nutritional needs are met without placing additional stress on the digestive system, which may be less efficient in such critically ill infants [11].

6. *Inborn errors of metabolism*: Certain genetic disorders, known as inborn errors of metabolism, may impair the body's ability to process specific nutrients or metabolites. These disorders can interfere with normal feeding or nutrient absorption, requiring individualized PN formulations to provide the neonate with the appropriate balance of nutrients while avoiding metabolic imbalances [6].

7. *Prolonged fasting or NPO status*: Neonates undergoing major surgeries, diagnostic procedures, or treatments that require prolonged fasting or nothing by mouth (NPO) status are at risk of inadequate nutrition. PN is initiated in these cases to prevent malnutrition and ensure adequate nutrient intake during the period of fasting or medical intervention [6].

3.2 Clinical scenarios necessitating parenteral nutrition

In the NICU, a variety of clinical scenarios may lead to the decision to initiate PN [12]. The following are examples of situations in which PN may be required:

- *Postoperative recovery*: After major surgical procedures such as cardiac surgery, abdominal surgery, or corrective surgeries for congenital anomalies, neonates often require PN while recovering and regaining the ability to tolerate enteral feeds [11].

- *Infections*: Critical infections, such as sepsis or meningitis, can increase metabolic demands and lead to impaired gut function. PN ensures that neonates maintain nutritional support during the acute phase of illness [13].

- *Chronic illnesses*: Neonates with chronic conditions, such as chronic lung disease of prematurity or cystic fibrosis, may experience difficulty with feeding and nutrient absorption, making PN an essential tool for long-term nutritional support [14].

- *Intestinal failure*: Some neonates may experience intestinal failure, a condition in which the gut is unable to absorb sufficient nutrients despite appropriate medical management. PN is often required to support these infants until their intestinal function improves or they can transition to enteral feeding. Intestinal failure (IF) is a well identified clinical condition, which is characterized by the reduction of functional gut capacity below the minimum needed for adequate digestion and absorption of nutrients for normal growth in children. Short bowel syndrome (SBS) is the leading cause of IF in neonates, infants, and young children [8].

3.3 Indications for starting neonatal parenteral nutrition (NICE guidelines 2024)

1. For preterm babies born before 31 + 0 weeks, start neonatal parenteral nutrition [6].

2. For preterm babies born at or after 31 + 0 weeks, start parenteral nutrition if sufficient progress is not made with enteral feeding in the first 72 hours after birth.

3. Start parenteral nutrition for preterm and term babies who are unlikely to establish sufficient enteral feeding, for example, babies with a congenital gut disorder, or a critical illness such as sepsis.

4. For preterm babies on enteral feeds, start parenteral nutrition if:

    - enteral feeds have to be stopped and it is unlikely they will be restarted within 48 hours

- enteral feeds have been stopped for more than 24 hours and there is unlikely to be sufficient progress with enteral feeding within a further 48 hours.

5. For term babies on enteral feeds, start parenteral nutrition if:

- enteral feeds have to be stopped and it is unlikely they will be restarted within 72 hours

- enteral feeds have been stopped for more than 48 hours and there is unlikely to be sufficient progress with enteral feeding within a further 48 hours.

4. Components of parenteral nutrition

Parenteral nutrition (PN) provides essential nutrients to neonates *via* intravenous infusion, bypassing the gastrointestinal tract. The components of PN are carefully formulated to meet the specific nutritional needs of neonates, particularly those who are premature, critically ill, or unable to tolerate enteral feeding. These components include macronutrients, micronutrients, fluids, and electrolytes, each playing a crucial role in the infant's growth, development, and metabolic function.

4.1 Macronutrients: Carbohydrates, proteins, and lipids

Macronutrients are the primary sources of energy for neonates and are essential for cellular growth, tissue repair, and overall development. The balance of carbohydrates, proteins, and lipids in PN must be carefully tailored to meet the individual needs of each neonate [15–18].

1. *Carbohydrates*: Carbohydrates are the primary source of energy in PN. Glucose, in the form of dextrose, is typically used as the carbohydrate source in neonatal PN formulations. It is metabolized by the body to produce energy, and glucose is vital for the brain and central nervous system development, especially in preterm infants who have high energy requirements. The concentration of glucose in PN must be carefully adjusted to avoid hyperglycemia or hypoglycemia, as neonates, particularly those with immature pancreatic function, are at risk for both.

   - *Energy source*: Glucose provides the necessary fuel for metabolic processes.

   - *Regulation*: Blood glucose levels need to be monitored regularly to ensure proper metabolic balance.

2. *Proteins*: Protein is essential for growth, tissue repair, immune function, and enzyme synthesis. In PN, amino acids, the building blocks of proteins, are provided to support the neonate's rapid development. The composition of amino acids in neonatal PN is designed to mimic human breast milk, providing essential amino acids that support protein synthesis and nitrogen balance.

- *Amino acids*: Essential amino acids like leucine, valine, and isoleucine are crucial for optimal growth.

- o Current amino acid solutions used in parenteral nutrition are designed based on three distinct methodologies. The first approach models the amino acid mixture after the composition of egg protein, primarily for adult use. This method was later adapted for neonates, but instead of egg protein, it was based on the amino acid profile of human milk, which is considered the ideal protein source for infants fed enterally. This approach assumes that the splanchnic bed (comprising the gut and liver) absorbs and metabolizes all enterally delivered amino acids uniformly and that all consumed amino acids reach the bloodstream—a notion that has been challenged by various studies. The second approach involves using the amino acid composition of cord blood. This commercially available solution is now widely utilized in Neonatal Intensive Care Units across North America and Europe. The third approach employs computer modeling to predict the plasma amino acid response to parenteral amino acid administration. A pediatric amino acid solution based on this model has been developed and is commonly used in NICUs in the United States. While this method assumes that optimal plasma amino acid concentrations are known, it does not account for the rates at which amino acids enter and exit the plasma pool [19].

- *Nitrogen balance*: The provision of adequate protein is vital for maintaining nitrogen balance and promoting positive growth.

3. *Lipids*: Lipids, mainly in the form of triglycerides, are another key energy source in PN. They provide essential fatty acids, which are necessary for cell membrane integrity, hormone synthesis, and brain development. Lipid emulsions used in neonatal PN are typically derived from soybean oil, olive oil, or fish oil, each offering different fatty acid profiles. Lipid solutions help reduce the risk of developing hypoglycemia, as they provide a steady source of calories over time [16].

- *Essential fatty acids*: Lipids provide omega-3 and omega-6 fatty acids, essential for brain and retinal development.

- *Energy storage*: Lipids provide a dense source of energy, important for neonates with high energy requirements.

4.2 Micronutrients: Vitamins, minerals, and trace elements

Micronutrients, including vitamins, minerals, and trace elements, are required in small amounts but are critical for metabolic processes, immune function, and growth. These nutrients must be carefully balanced in PN to prevent deficiencies or toxicities, as the immature liver and kidneys of neonates may have limited capacity to metabolize excess amounts [18].

1. *Vitamins*: Vitamins are essential for a wide range of physiological processes, including bone health, immune function, and the prevention of oxidative damage. In neonatal PN, the vitamins typically included are:

   - *Fat-soluble vitamins*: Vitamin A, D, E, and K, which are important for vision, bone health, antioxidant protection, and blood clotting, respectively.

- *Water-soluble vitamins*: Vitamin C, B vitamins (e.g., B12, folic acid, and thiamine), which support immune function, red blood cell formation, and energy metabolism.

2. *Minerals*: Minerals are vital for maintaining fluid balance, bone formation, and enzyme function. Commonly included minerals in PN for neonates are:

    - *Calcium and phosphorus*: Important for bone mineralization and growth.

    - *Magnesium*: Essential for muscle and nerve function.

    - *Sodium, potassium, chloride*: Electrolytes that help maintain acid-base balance, osmotic pressure, and fluid balance.

3. *Trace elements*: Trace elements such as zinc, copper, selenium, and manganese are needed in minute quantities but play important roles in enzyme function, growth, and immunity. These are included in PN formulations to prevent deficiencies, which can lead to delayed growth and immune dysfunction.

    - *Zinc*: Important for wound healing and immune function.

    - *Copper*: Necessary for iron metabolism and the formation of red blood cells.

    - *Selenium*: Acts as an antioxidant, protecting cells from oxidative damage.

4.3 Fluid and electrolyte management

Fluid and electrolyte balance is a critical component of neonatal PN, as neonates are highly sensitive to fluctuations in hydration status [20]. Both excess and deficiency of fluids and electrolytes can lead to serious complications, including dehydration, overhydration, or electrolyte imbalances. The formulation of PN must account for the neonate's specific fluid and electrolyte needs, which can vary based on their weight, age, and clinical condition.

It is important to note that electrolyte imbalances alone are not indication to start PN. PN is not recommended as the first line management of electrolyte imbalances. Instead, electrolyte imbalance should be addressed first through appropriate fluid management, followed by the initiation of parenteral nutrition if there is a valid indication.

- *Fluid needs*: The total volume of fluids is adjusted based on the neonate's age, weight, and clinical condition. It is crucial to provide the right amount of fluid to avoid fluid overload, especially in preterm infants with immature kidneys.

Table 1 shows details of fluid requirement in normal neonates based on birth weight and postnatal age [20].

- *Electrolyte requirements*: Sodium, potassium, calcium, and magnesium are carefully included in the PN formulation to maintain normal cellular and metabolic function, as well as to support growth and development.

Day of Life	<1000 g	1001–1500 g	1501–2000 g	>2500 g
Day 1	100–120 ml	80–100 ml	60–80 ml	50–70 ml
Day 2	120–150 ml	110–130 ml	90–110 ml	80–100 ml
Day 3	150–170 ml	140–160 ml	120–140 ml	100–120 ml
Day 4	180–200 ml	160–180 ml	140–160 ml	130–150 ml
Day 5 onwards	180–200 ml	170–200 ml	150–180 ml	140–160 ml

Table 1.
Details of fluid requirement in normal neonates based on birth weight and postnatal age.

5. Initiating and monitoring parenteral nutrition

The successful initiation and monitoring of parenteral nutrition (PN) in neonates require careful planning, individualized dosing, and ongoing assessment to ensure that the neonate receives adequate nutrition while minimizing the risks of complications. The initiation process must take into account the neonate's clinical condition, gestational age, and specific nutritional needs, as well as the ability to tolerate PN. Monitoring ensures that the neonate's growth, metabolic status, and response to PN are tracked, allowing for timely adjustments to the nutritional regimen [3, 4, 21].

5.1 Formulation and prescription of parenteral nutrition

The formulation of PN is customized for each neonate based on several factors, including gestational age, postnatal age, weight, and clinical condition [18]. The goal is to provide a balance of macronutrients (carbohydrates, proteins, and lipids), micronutrients (vitamins and minerals), and electrolytes while avoiding complications such as hyperglycemia, electrolyte imbalances, or nutrient deficiencies.

1. *Initial formulation* For neonates, especially preterm infants, PN is typically initiated at lower doses and gradually increased as the infant stabilizes. Early PN support, often within the first 24 hours of life, is recommended to meet the high energy demands of rapidly growing neonates. The formulation includes the following components:

    - *Carbohydrates*: Dextrose (glucose) is the primary source of energy. The initial dextrose infusion rate is often set at a conservative rate (e.g., 4–6 mg/kg/min) and can be increased as the neonate tolerates.

    - *Proteins*: Amino acids are included to support growth and nitrogen balance. The initial protein dose is typically lower and is gradually increased to meet the neonate's growing needs [22].

        - "The amino acid composition of breastmilk uniquely meets the needs of healthy term infants; bovine protein contains a different balance of amino acids and needs to be provided in a higher dose to compensate for relative shortage of certain (conditionally) essential amino acid. The optimal composition of amino acids in PN has not been widely studied and it remains unclear what the reference ranges for plasma amino acids should be, particularly because fetal blood concentrations differ from healthy infants ex-utero. 11 Several PN studies show a wide range of concentrations for both essential and non-essential amino acids, raising the possibility that certain amino acids may be provided in excess and could be neuro-toxic, or conversely that they may be rate limiting for lean mass accretion. Regardless of the optimal plasma amino acid profile, currently available PN solutions will not provide a 'protein quality' as high as human milk protein. In addition, most studies do not consider the hydration factor of amino acids in PN, thereby overestimating true protein intakes. Around 15% of the weight of an individual amino acid in PN is lost in the form of water once polymers are formed as protein. Therefore, a higher intake of amino acids (as nitrogen) in PN might be needed to match the quality and quantity of protein provided by human milk" [22].

- *Lipids*: Lipid emulsions provide essential fatty acids and additional caloric support. Lipid infusion rates should be started at low levels and adjusted based on the neonate's tolerance.

- *Electrolytes*:

  o It is essential to start sodium and potassium from the beginning at day one with the recommended dose for age once the patient's diuresis and renal function are confirmed to be normal otherwise it should be adjusted accordingly.

  o "Historically, there were concerns that provision of sodium in the first few postnatal days may impair the early water loss needed as extracellular fluid volume contracts after birth. Excess sodium and fluid intakes in this period may worsen respiratory function. However, sodium-free PN restricts the ability to provide disodium-glycerophosphate, the contemporary primary formulation of parenteral phosphate. Similarly, the incidence of early hypokalaemia can be reduced by providing higher intakes of potassium" [22].

  o Magnesium, calcium, and phosphorus initiation should be on the first day and as soon as possible especially for preterm newborns. However, according to some experts, their initiation can be delayed in some cases for up to 2–3 days; however, this is a controversial point, and the decision can vary depending on the patient's condition.

  o The initial dose of electrolytes will be different from patient to patient according to his blood levels, fluid status, and many factors.

Table 2 shows a guide to the electrolytes' doses in general.

2. *Adjusting formulation over time* As the neonate's clinical condition improves or stabilizes, the PN formulation may be adjusted to meet their evolving nutritional requirements. Nutritional needs are influenced by factors such as weight gain, growth velocity, and clinical progress. The formulation may need to be altered to [1]:

Electrolyte	Preterm neonates	Infants/children
Sodium	2–5 mEq/kg/day	2–5 mEq/kg/day
Potassium	2–4 mEq/kg/day	2–4 mEq/kg/day
Calcium	2–4 mEq/kg/day	0.5–4 mEq/kg/day
Phosphorus	1–2 mmol/kg/day	0.5–2 mmol/kg/day
Magnesium	0.3–0.5 mEq/kg/day	0.3–0.5 mEq/kg/day

Source: Ref. [23].

Table 2.
A guide to the electrolytes' doses in general.

	Initiation		Advance By		Goals	
	Preterm	Term	Preterm	Term	Preterm	Term
Protein (g/kg/d)	1–3 (3–4 max)	2.5–3	—	—	3–4	2.5–3
Dextrose (mg/kg/min)	6–8	6–8	1–2	1–2	10–14 (max 14–18)	10–14 (max 14–18)
ILE (g/kg/d)	0.5–1	0.5–1	0.5–1	0.5–1	3 (max 0.15 g/kg/h)	2.5–3 (max 0.15 g/kg/h)

Table 3.
Recommended parenteral intakes of different nutrients in early parenteral nutrition for neonates (macronutrients).

- Increase protein intake to support tissue repair and growth.
- Adjust the ratio of lipids and carbohydrates based on the neonate's energy needs and tolerance.
- Include additional micronutrients, particularly in cases of specific deficiencies or clinical conditions (e.g., metabolic disorders).

Tables 3 and **4** show recommended parenteral intakes of different nutrients in early parenteral nutrition for neonates:

5.2 Monitoring growth and metabolic parameters

Regular monitoring is essential to assess how well the neonate is responding to PN and to detect early signs of complications [6]. Key parameters to monitor include growth, metabolic markers, and organ function [24].

1. *Growth monitoring* Growth is a primary indicator of the effectiveness of PN. The following measures are used to assess growth:

- *Weight gain*: Monitoring weight gain is critical in assessing whether the neonate is receiving adequate nutrition. Ideally, neonates should gain weight steadily, although preterm infants may experience slower growth in the early weeks.

Component	Initial amount	Target amount
Total energy	45–60 kcal/kg/day	80–90 kcal/kg/day
Nonprotein energy	35–45 kcal/kg/day	>65 kcal/kg/day
Amino acid	1.5–2.5 g/kg/day	2.5–3.5 g/kg/day
		OR Weight-based dosing:
		<1000 g: 2.5–3.5 g/kg/day
		≥1000 to <1500 g: 3.0–3.5 g/kg/day
		≥1500 to 2000 g: 3 g/kg/day
Lipid	0–1 g/kg/day	2–3 g/kg/day
Sodium	2–4 mEq/kg/day	3–5 mEq/kg/day *OR* 69–115 mg/kg/day
Potassium	2–4 mEq/kg/day	2–3 mEq/kg/day *OR* 78–117 mg/kg/day
Calcium	25–50 mg/kg/day	65–100 mg/kg/day
Magnesium	0–3 mg/kg/day	4.3–10 mg/kg/day
Phosphorus	None	50–80 mg/kg/day
Iron	None	0.0–0.25 mg/kg/day
Zinc	None	0.4 mg/kg/day
Copper	None	40 mcg/kg/day
Selenium	None	1.5–4.5 mcg/kg/day
Manganese	None	1 mcg/kg/day
Chromium	None	0.05–0.3 mcg/kg/day
Carnitine	None	10 mg/kg/day
Vitamin A	None	700–1500 IU/kg/day
Vitamin D	None	40–160 IU/kg/day
Vitamin E	None	2.8–3.5 IU/kg/day
Vitamin K	None	10 mcg/kg/day
Vitamin C	None	15–25 mg/kg/day
Vitamin B1 (thiamine)	None	200–350 mcg/kg/day
Vitamin B2 (riboflavin)	None	150–200 mcg/kg/day
Vitamin B3 (niacin)	None	4.0–6.8 mg/kg/day
Vitamin B5 (pantothenate)	None	1–2 mg/kg/day
Vitamin B6 (pyridoxine)	None	150–200 mcg/kg/day
Vitamin B7 (biotin)	None	5–8 mcg/kg/day
Vitamin B9 (folic acid)	None	56 mcg/kg/day
Vitamin B12 (cobalamin)	None	0.3 mcg/kg/day

Source: Ref. [23].

Table 4.
Recommended parenteral intakes of different nutrients in early parenteral nutrition for neonates (macronutrients and micronutrients).

- *Length and head circumference*: These growth parameters are also monitored, particularly in preterm and VLBW (very low birth weight) infants, to ensure they are following normal growth patterns.

2. *Metabolic monitoring* Metabolic parameters are regularly assessed to detect any imbalances or adverse effects related to PN:

- *Blood glucose levels*: Regular monitoring of blood glucose is essential to detect and prevent hyperglycemia or hypoglycemia, which are common complications in neonates receiving PN.

- *Electrolyte levels*: Monitoring sodium, potassium, calcium, magnesium, and phosphate levels is necessary to prevent and manage electrolyte disturbances.

- *Liver function*: Liver enzymes (such as ALT, AST, and bilirubin) are monitored to detect signs of hepatic dysfunction or cholestasis, which can be complications of long-term PN use [13].

- *Renal function*: Kidney function should be regularly assessed through serum creatinine and urine output to ensure that the neonate's kidneys are handling the fluid and electrolyte load appropriately.

- *Serum triglycerides*: Measure serum triglycerides daily while increasing the parenteral nutrition lipid dosage, and weekly after reaching a maintenance intravenous lipid dosage. Measure serum triglycerides more frequently, but not more than once a day, if the level is elevated or if the preterm or term baby is at risk of hypertriglyceridaemia, for example, if the baby is critically ill or has a lipaemic blood sample. Ongoing serum triglyceride monitoring may not be needed for stable preterm or term babies transitioning from parenteral nutrition to enteral nutrition [25].

3. *Nutrient imbalance detection* Frequent testing of blood work is necessary to detect nutrient imbalances. For example, insufficient phosphate levels can lead to metabolic bone disease, while excessive glucose intake can lead to hyperglycemia. Regular blood tests help clinicians adjust the PN formula to correct any imbalances before they result in complications [6].

Test	First 3–7 days	Thereafter
Electrolytes, BUN, HCO_3, Creatinine	Daily or as needed	Once or twice a week
Ca, PO_4, Mg, bilirubin, albumin	As needed	Once a week
Triglyceride	24 hours after each increase	Once a week or when sick
Blood glucose	4–6 hourly	Once or twice a day
Liver function test including alkaline phosphatase	As needed	Once weekly or fortnightly

Source: Ref. [6].

Table 5.
How frequent biochemical monitoring parameters should be checked during PN.

Table 5 shows how frequent biochemical monitoring parameters should be checked during PN.

5.3 Adjusting parenteral nutrition based on clinical progress

As the neonate's condition evolves, PN needs to be adjusted accordingly [2]. Clinical progress can be influenced by the neonate's ability to tolerate the PN, overall metabolic stability, and the resolution of any underlying medical conditions. Key factors in adjusting PN include:

1. *Tolerating higher volumes and concentrations*: As the neonate stabilizes, the volume and concentration of PN can be increased to meet growing nutritional needs. This includes increasing the calorie density, protein intake, and other micronutrients.

2. *Transitioning to enteral feeds*: As the neonate's gastrointestinal system matures or heals, enteral feeding may be introduced. The transition from PN to enteral feeding involves gradually decreasing the PN while slowly increasing the amount of enteral nutrition, monitoring for signs of feeding intolerance.

3. *Handling complications*: Any complications, such as infection, metabolic disturbances, or feeding intolerance, must be managed promptly. PN should be adjusted to address these issues, such as reducing glucose in cases of hyperglycemia or adding additional lipids to provide better energy balance.

6. Challenges and complications of parenteral nutrition

While parenteral nutrition (PN) is a vital intervention for neonates who cannot tolerate enteral feeding, its use in the neonatal intensive care unit (NICU) is associated with several challenges and potential complications. These complications can arise from the inherent risks of intravenous feeding, long-term use, and the complex needs of neonates, particularly those who are preterm or critically ill [26].

6.1 Metabolic complications

Metabolic disturbances are among the most common complications of PN, and they can significantly impact the neonate's health and recovery [3, 5, 10]. These complications can arise from the administration of excess or insufficient nutrients, inappropriate fluid balance, or the neonate's immature metabolic capacity.

1. *Hyperglycemia*: Hyperglycemia, or elevated blood glucose levels, is one of the most frequent metabolic complications in neonates receiving PN. Preterm infants, particularly those with low birth weight, are at a higher risk due to their immature insulin regulation and limited pancreatic function. Hyperglycemia can lead to adverse outcomes such as electrolyte disturbances, osmotic diuresis, dehydration, and an increased risk of infections.

   - *Management*: Tight blood glucose monitoring is essential. Insulin may be required to manage hyperglycemia, and the glucose infusion rate should be adjusted to avoid excessive dextrose administration.

  - Insulin is rarely required to manage hyperglycemia during parenteral nutrition (PN) and should be used only in special circumstances. Due to the heightened risk of hypoglycemia in neonates, even standard insulin doses should generally be avoided for PN-associated hyperglycemia unless clinically justified.

2. *Hypoglycemia*: Hypoglycemia, or low blood glucose levels, can occur when PN formulations contain inadequate carbohydrates or if the neonate's glucose utilization exceeds the amount provided. It is particularly concerning in very low birth weight (VLBW) and extremely low birth weight (ELBW) infants who have limited glycogen stores.

    - *Management*: Blood glucose levels should be monitored frequently. If hypoglycemia is detected, the PN formulation may be adjusted by increasing glucose concentration, and feeding protocols may be adapted to ensure consistent glucose supply.

3. *Electrolyte imbalances*: PN can lead to various electrolyte imbalances, including disturbances in sodium, potassium, calcium, and phosphate levels. These imbalances can result from incorrect formulation, changes in fluid balance, or the neonate's immature renal function, which may impair their ability to regulate electrolytes effectively.

    - *Management*: Regular monitoring of electrolyte levels is essential, and adjustments to the PN formulation may be required. For example, phosphate supplementation is often necessary for neonates on long-term PN, as they are at risk for developing hypophosphatemia.

4. *Metabolic bone disease*: Neonates receiving long-term PN are at risk for developing metabolic bone disease, a condition characterized by low bone mineral density, increased bone fragility, and growth retardation. This can be caused by insufficient calcium and phosphate intake, as well as altered vitamin D metabolism.

    - *Management*: Monitoring of calcium and phosphate levels and the inclusion of vitamin D in the PN formulation is crucial to prevent or treat metabolic bone disease. In some cases, the administration of additional calcium and phosphate may be required.

5. *Refeeding Syndrome*: It is a life-threatening complication that can occur in neonates receiving parenteral nutrition, particularly after prolonged periods of malnutrition. The syndrome arises when the sudden reintroduction of carbohydrates triggers a surge in insulin, leading to an abrupt intracellular shift of key electrolytes—especially phosphorus, potassium, and magnesium—which are critical for cellular function. This rapid change can precipitate severe hypophosphatemia, hypokalemia, and hypomagnesemia, resulting in cardiac, respiratory, and neurological complications. Given the delicate metabolic balance in neonates, careful monitoring and gradual advancement of nutritional support are essential to prevent these dangerous electrolyte imbalances and ensure safe recovery.

6.2 Infection risks and catheter management

Infection is a significant risk for neonates receiving PN, particularly those with central venous catheters (CVCs) or peripherally inserted central catheters (PICCs) used for the administration of PN [27, 28]. These catheters are prone to infections, including catheter-related bloodstream infections (CRBSIs), which can lead to sepsis and other life-threatening complications [29].

1. *Catheter-related bloodstream infections (CRBSIs)*: CRBSIs occur when bacteria or fungi colonize the catheter and enter the bloodstream, leading to systemic infections. These infections are a major concern for neonates receiving PN, as they can result in significant morbidity and mortality.

   - *Management*: Strict adherence to sterile techniques during catheter insertion and maintenance is essential. Prophylactic antibiotics may be considered in high-risk infants, and catheter care protocols must be followed rigorously to prevent infection. In the case of suspected CRBSI, prompt removal of the catheter and initiation of appropriate antimicrobial therapy are required.

2. *Catheter occlusion and thrombosis*: Catheter occlusion can occur due to the formation of clots or the accumulation of lipids or other substances within the catheter. This can disrupt the administration of PN and lead to complications such as venous thrombosis or poor nutritional support.

   - *Management*: Regular flushing of the catheter with saline or heparinized saline can help prevent occlusions. If an occlusion occurs, appropriate interventions, such as fibrinolytic therapy or catheter replacement, may be necessary.

6.3 Long-term effects of prolonged parenteral nutrition

While PN is a lifesaving therapy for neonates in the short term, prolonged use can lead to significant long-term complications. These can affect multiple organ systems and require ongoing management to minimize negative outcomes [8, 13, 29–32].

1. *Intestinal failure and dependence on PN:* Prolonged PN use in neonates with conditions such as short bowel syndrome or necrotizing enterocolitis (NEC) can result in intestinal failure, where the gastrointestinal tract is unable to absorb adequate nutrients. These neonates may become dependent on PN for extended periods, and some may require long-term or even lifelong PN support.

   - *Management*: Intestinal rehabilitation strategies, including enteral feeding (as tolerated) and growth factors such as GLP-2[1], are often employed to improve gastrointestinal function and reduce reliance on PN.

[1] The recombinant analogue of human glucagon-like peptide-2 (GLP-2) teduglutide (Gattex_, Revestive_) is a novel therapeutic option for SBS. GLP-2 is a naturally occurring hormone regulating the growth, proliferation, and maintenance of cells in the gastrointestinal tract [33].

2. *Liver dysfunction and cholestasis:* Prolonged PN use can lead to liver dysfunction, particularly cholestasis, a condition characterized by impaired bile flow and the accumulation of bile acids in the liver. Cholestasis is a common complication in neonates receiving long-term PN and can lead to liver damage and failure if left untreated.

    - *Management*: Early detection of cholestasis is important. Management strategies include optimizing the PN formula, introducing enteral feeds as soon as possible, and using medications such as ursodeoxycholic acid to promote bile flow. In severe cases, liver transplantation may be considered; however, liver failure requiring transplantation is extremely rare, liver failure is typically reversible, and it can often be resolved by discontinuing PN.

3. *Metabolic adaptation and growth challenges:* Long-term PN can impact the neonate's ability to grow at an optimal rate, particularly if there are nutrient imbalances or complications such as metabolic bone disease. Neonates with complex medical conditions or who have been on prolonged PN may experience delayed or impaired growth.

    - *Management*: Close monitoring of growth parameters, including weight gain, head circumference, and length, is essential. Adjusting the PN formula to meet the infant's increasing energy needs and addressing any nutrient deficiencies is critical to support ongoing growth and development.

7. Transitioning from parenteral to enteral nutrition

Transitioning from parenteral nutrition (PN) to enteral nutrition is a crucial process for neonates, particularly those in the neonatal intensive care unit (NICU) who have been on prolonged PN. This transition represents a shift from intravenous feeding to gastrointestinal feeding, which is essential for the neonate's development and recovery. The ability to tolerate enteral nutrition is an important milestone, signaling improved gastrointestinal function and readiness for a more physiological mode of feeding.

The process of transitioning from PN to enteral nutrition must be carefully managed to ensure that the neonate receives adequate nutrition while avoiding complications such as feeding intolerance, aspiration, or fluid imbalances.

7.1 Indicators for weaning off parenteral nutrition

The decision to begin transitioning from PN to enteral feeding depends on several clinical and physiological factors that suggest the neonate's gastrointestinal system is ready to handle enteral nutrition. Key indicators include [2, 3]:

1. *Improved gastrointestinal function*: Neonates must demonstrate sufficient gastrointestinal motility and digestive enzyme activity to tolerate enteral feeding. Signs that suggest the neonate's gastrointestinal system is functional include:

- Adequate bowel sounds and the ability to pass stool.
- Absence of abdominal distension or discomfort.
- Tolerance to small volumes of enteral feeds without signs of feeding intolerance, such as vomiting, diarrhea, or bloating.

2. *Clinical stability and weight gain*: The neonate's overall clinical condition must be stable, with no ongoing signs of acute illness or metabolic instability. Additionally, the infant should be showing consistent weight gain, indicating that growth can be supported by enteral nutrition.

   - Stable vital signs (e.g., temperature, heart rate, blood pressure).
   - Improved feeding tolerance and consistent weight gain are key signs that PN may be reduced.

3. *Absence of major medical conditions*: Neonates with certain medical conditions, such as necrotizing enterocolitis (NEC), significant gastrointestinal malformations, or severe feeding difficulties, may require a prolonged period of PN. If these conditions have resolved or are under control, the transition to enteral feeding can be considered.

4. *Ability to tolerate initial enteral feeds*: When enteral feeding is first introduced, the neonate must demonstrate the ability to tolerate the feeds without significant clinical issues. This includes:

   - Minimal residual stomach content or vomiting.
   - The absence of significant gastrointestinal discomfort.

7.2 Strategies for introducing enteral feeds

The introduction of enteral nutrition is a gradual process that requires careful monitoring and adjustment. Several strategies can help ensure that this transition is successful [1, 34]:

1. *Gradual introduction of small volumes*: Enteral feeding is typically started with small volumes (e.g., 5–10 mL every few hours) of an appropriate formula or breast milk. These feeds are introduced slowly to assess the neonate's tolerance and allow the gastrointestinal system to adapt.

   - Initially, only a small proportion of the neonate's nutritional needs will be met through enteral feeding.
   - Over time, the volume of enteral feeds is gradually increased, while PN volumes are decreased.

2. *Monitoring for feeding intolerance*: During the transition, it is critical to monitor the neonate for signs of feeding intolerance. This can include:

- *Vomiting, diarrhea, and abdominal distension*: These symptoms may indicate intolerance to the enteral feeds or the need for adjustments in the feeding protocol.

- *Signs of aspiration*: Aspiration can occur if the neonate inhales milk or formula into the lungs, which can lead to respiratory distress or pneumonia.

  If feeding intolerance is observed, the volume of enteral feeds should be reduced, and the feed rate should be slowed or paused temporarily. Gradual reintroduction may be necessary once symptoms resolve.

3. *Balanced feeding approach*: A balanced approach involves carefully balancing enteral and parenteral feeds during the transition. The goal is to ensure that the neonate's nutritional needs are met while preventing overloading the gastrointestinal system. As enteral feeds increase, PN is gradually tapered to avoid overfeeding and the risk of metabolic disturbances.

4. *Use of human milk or fortified formula*: Whenever possible, breast milk should be used as the primary source of enteral nutrition. Breast milk provides optimal nutrition, including essential antibodies, and supports gastrointestinal maturation. Donor-milk can be used as an alternative in the absence of the infant's own maternal breast milk. If breast milk is unavailable, a nutritionally balanced preterm formula or fortified formula may be used to meet the neonate's nutritional needs.

   - *Fortification*: In preterm infants or those with increased nutritional needs, breast milk may be fortified with additional calories, proteins, or micronutrients to support growth and development.

7.3 Ongoing monitoring during transition

Close monitoring is essential throughout the transition process to ensure that the neonate is adapting to enteral feeds and that nutritional goals are being met. Key aspects of monitoring include [6, 13]:

1. *Growth parameters*: Regularly monitoring the neonate's weight, length, and head circumference is essential to ensure that growth is on track as enteral feeds are introduced. Any signs of poor growth should prompt an evaluation of feeding tolerance and adjustments to the nutritional regimen.

2. *Hydration and electrolyte balance*: The transition to enteral feeding can affect fluid balance and electrolyte levels, so regular monitoring of hydration status and electrolytes is crucial. This includes assessing:

   - *Urine output*: Adequate urine output is a sign of proper hydration.

   - *Electrolyte levels*: Sodium, potassium, and calcium should be monitored to avoid imbalances.

3. *Nutritional adequacy*: As enteral feeding is introduced, it is essential to assess whether the neonate is receiving adequate nutrition. Laboratory tests, such as serum glucose, protein, and electrolyte levels, should be checked regularly to detect any early signs of nutrient deficiencies or imbalances.

- *Blood glucose*: Ensure that glucose levels remain stable as enteral feeds increase and PN decreases.

- *Albumin and prealbumin*: These protein markers may be assessed to evaluate nutritional status and protein intake.

4. *Transition planning and coordination*: Successful transition from PN to enteral nutrition requires careful planning and coordination among the healthcare team. Multidisciplinary collaboration between neonatologists, dietitians, nurses, and pharmacists ensures that feeding protocols are tailored to the individual neonate's needs. Family involvement in the feeding process is also important to support feeding practices and ensure smooth discharge planning.

8. Conclusion

Parenteral nutrition (PN) is a critical intervention in neonatal intensive care units, providing essential nutrients to neonates who cannot tolerate enteral feeding. It serves as a lifeline for preterm and critically ill infants, ensuring adequate growth, metabolic stability, and improved health outcomes. The formulation and administration of PN require careful customization to meet the unique needs of each neonate, balancing macronutrients, micronutrients, and fluids while minimizing risks.

Despite its lifesaving benefits, PN is associated with challenges, including complications like hyperglycemia, electrolyte imbalances, and catheter-related infections. Therefore, monitoring and individualized adjustments are essential to optimize its effectiveness and minimize adverse effects. Transitioning from PN to enteral feeding remains a crucial goal, requiring a gradual, well-monitored approach to ensure gastrointestinal adaptation and sustained growth.

Acknowledgements

The author acknowledges the use of [ChatGPT] for language polishing and editing assistance in preparing this manuscript. The author also confirms that the AI tool was used solely for improving the clarity and readability of the text, and full responsibility for the content, accuracy, and integrity of the manuscript remains with the author.

Author details

Hossam A. Elgnainy
Cairo University Specialized Pediatric Hospital, Cairo, Egypt

*Address all correspondence to: helgnainy@gmail.com

References

[1] Groh-Wargo S, Barr SM. Parenteral Nutrition. Clinics in Perinatology. 2022;**49**(2):355-379. DOI: 10.1016/j.clp.2022.02.002

[2] Bolisetty S. Parenteral Nutrition in Newborns. Sydney: South Eastern Sydney Local Health District (SESLHD); 2018. Available from: https://www.seslhd.health.nsw.gov.au/sites/default/files/migration/RHW/Newborn_Care/Guidelines/Medical/nccparenteralnutrition.pdf

[3] Robinson DT, Calkins KL, Chen Y, Cober MP, Falciglia GH, Church DD, et al. Guidelines for parenteral nutrition in preterm infants: The American Society for Parenteral and Enteral Nutrition. JPEN Journal of Parenteral and Enteral Nutrition. 2023;**47**(7):830-858. DOI: 10.1002/jpen.2550. Epub 2023 Aug 23. Erratum in: JPEN J Parenter Enteral Nutr. Feb 2024;**48**(2):242-244. DOI: 10.1002/jpen.2582

[4] American Society for Parenteral and Enteral Nutrition. Appropriate Dosing for Parenteral Nutrition: ASPEN Recommendations. American Society for Parenteral and Enteral Nutrition; 2019. Available from: https://nutritioncare.org/wp-content/uploads/2024/12/Appropriate-Dosing-for-PN.pdf

[5] Chacham S, Pasi R, Chegondi M, Ahmad N, Mohanty SB. Metabolic bone disease in premature neonates: An unmet challenge. Journal of Clinical Research in Pediatric Endocrinology. 2020;**12**(4):332-339. DOI: 10.4274/jcrpe.galenos.2019.2019.0091. Epub 2019 Nov 1

[6] National Institute for Health and Care Excellence (NICE). Neonatal Parenteral Nutrition. London: NICE; 2020. Available from: https://www.nice.org.uk/guidance/ng154/resources/neonatal-parenteral-nutrition-pdf-66141840283333

[7] Pybus R, Puntis JW. Parenteral nutrition. Archives of Disease in Childhood. 1 Sep 2021;**106**(9):921-922. Available from: https://adc.bmj.com/content/106/9/921

[8] Bering J, DiBaise JK. Short bowel syndrome: Complications and management. Nutrition in Clinical Practice. 2023;**38**(Suppl. 1):S46-S58. DOI: 10.1002/ncp.10978

[9] Ou J, Courtney CM, Steinberger AE, Tecos ME, Warner BW. Nutrition in necrotizing enterocolitis and following intestinal resection. Nutrients. 2020;**12**(2):520. DOI: 10.3390/nu12020520

[10] Balasundaram P, Dumpa V. Neonatal hyperglycemia. In: StatPearls. StatPearls Publishing; 2023. Available from: https://www.ncbi.nlm.nih.gov/books/NBK567769/

[11] Mills KI, Kim JH, Fogg K, Goldshtrom N, Graham EM, Kataria-Hale J, et al. Nutritional considerations for the neonate with congenital heart disease. Pediatrics. 2022;**150**(Suppl. 2):e2022056415G. DOI: 10.1542/peds.2022-056415G

[12] Yoshida T, Goya H, Iida N, Arakaki M, Sanabe N, Nakanishi K. Early parenteral nutrition in neonates with congenital diaphragmatic hernia. Pediatrics International. Feb 2020;**62**(2):200-205. Available from: https://onlinelibrary.wiley.com/doi/full/10.1111/ped.14083

[13] Wang YS, Shen W, Yang Q, Lin R, Tang LX, Bai RM, et al. Analysis of

risk factors for parenteral nutrition-associated cholestasis in preterm infants: A multicenter observational study. BMC Pediatrics. 2023;**23**(1):250. DOI: 10.1186/s12887-023-04068-0. Erratum in: BMC Pediatr. 17 Jun 2023;**23**(1):305. DOI: 10.1186/s12887-023-04116-9

[14] Luca AC, Miron IC, Mîndru DE, Curpăn AȘ, Stan RC, Țarcă E, et al. Optimal nutrition parameters for neonates and infants with congenital heart disease. Nutrients. 2022;**14**(8):1671. DOI: 10.3390/nu14081671

[15] Carnielli VP, Correani A, Giretti I, D'Ascenzo R, Bellagamba MP, Burattini I, et al. Practice of parenteral Nutrition in preterm infants. World Review of Nutrition and Dietetics. 1 Jan 2021;**122**:198-211. Available from: https://pubmed.ncbi.nlm.nih.gov/34352767/

[16] Chan AP, Rostas S, Rogers S, Martin CR, Calkins KL. Parenteral Nutrition in the neonatal intensive care unit: Intravenous lipid emulsions. Clinics in Perinatology. 1 Sep 2023;**50**(3):575-589. Available from: https://pubmed.ncbi.nlm.nih.gov/37536765/

[17] Karthigesu K, Bertolo RF, Brown RJ. Parenteral nutrition and oxidant load in neonates. Nutrients. 30 Jul 2021;**13**(8):2631. Available from: https://www.mdpi.com/2072-6643/13/8/2631

[18] Rizzo V, Capozza M, Panza R, Laforgia N, Baldassarre ME. Macronutrients and micronutrients in parenteral nutrition for preterm newborns: A narrative review. Nutrients. 2022;**14**(7):1530. DOI: 10.3390/nu14071530

[19] Prolla I, Tomlinson C, Pencharz PB, Porto B, Elango R, Courtney-Martin G. Amino acid requirements of total parenteral nutrition (TPN) fed neonates: A narrative review of current knowledge and the basis for a new amino acid solution in neonatal nutrition. Pediatric Medicine. 2022;**5**. Available from: https://pm.amegroups.org/article/view/6123/html

[20] Mohanharjai M. Fluid and electrolyte concepts in new borns. Medical Journal, Armed Forces India. 2011;**58**(2):182

[21] Akour A, Gharaibeh L, El Khatib O, Hammour KA, AlTaher N, AbuRuz S, et al. Treatment-related problems in neonates receiving parenteral nutrition: Risk factors and implications for practice. BMC Pediatrics. 3 Jan 2024;**24**(1):4. Available from: https://bmcpediatr.biomedcentral.com/articles/10.1186/s12887-023-04477-1

[22] Embleton ND, van den Akker CH. Protein intakes for preterm infants, and the need for a multi-nutrient holistic approach. Pediatric Research. 2024;**1-3**. Available from: https://www.nature.com/articles/s41390-024-03453-4

[23] UpToDate. Neonatal Parenteral Nutrition. Waltham, MA: UpToDate; 2025. Available from: https://www.uptodate.com/contents/image?topicKey=PEDS%2F5026&search=neonatal+parenteral+nutrition&imageKey=PEDS%2F117237&rank=2%7E150&source=see_link

[24] Mihatsch W, Jiménez Varas MÁ, Diehl LL, Carnielli V, Schuler R, Gebauer C, et al. Systematic review on individualized versus standardized parenteral nutrition in preterm infants. Nutrients. 28 Feb 2023;**15**(5):1224. Available from: https://pubmed.ncbi.nlm.nih.gov/36904223/

[25] Deshpande GC, Cai W. Use of lipids in neonates requiring parenteral Nutrition. JPEN Journal of Parenteral

and Enteral Nutrition. 2020;**44**(Suppl. 1): S45-S54. DOI: 10.1002/jpen.1759

[26] da Silva JS, Seres DS, Sabino K, Adams SC, Berdahl GJ, Citty SW, et al. ASPEN consensus recommendations for refeeding syndrome. Nutrition in Clinical Practice. Apr 2020;**35**(2):178-195. Available from: https://pubmed.ncbi.nlm.nih.gov/32115791/

[27] Mays A, Ayers P, Monczka J, Cober MP. Safety in parenteral nutrition compounding. Nutrition in Clinical Practice. 2023;**38**(6):1253-1262. DOI: 10.1002/ncp.11064. Epub 2023 Aug 16

[28] Senterre T, van den Akker CHP, Domellof M, Saenz de Pipaon M, Arnell H, Tabbers M, et al. Safe and efficient practice of parenteral nutrition in neonates and children aged 0-18 years - the role of licensed multi-chamber bags. Clinical Nutrition. 2024;**43**(7):1696-1705. DOI: 10.1016/j.clnu.2024.05.023. Epub 2024 May 15

[29] Mirtallo J, Johnson D, Kumpf V. Safe practices for parenteral nutrition. JPEN, Journal of Parenteral and Enteral Nutrition. 1 Nov 2004;**28**(6):S39. Available from: https://pubmed.ncbi.nlm.nih.gov/15568296/

[30] Anne RP, Kadyada SP, Aradhya AS, Oleti TP. Ursodeoxycholic acid for preventing parenteral nutrition-associated cholestasis in neonates: A systematic review and meta-analysis. Fundamental and Clinical Pharmacology. 2024;**38**(4):685-694. DOI: 10.1111/fcp.12993. Epub 2024 Feb 11

[31] Guglielmi FW, Boggio-Bertinet D, Federico A, Forte GB, Guglielmi A, Loguercio C, et al. Total parenteral nutrition-related gastroenterological complications. Digestive and Liver Disease. 1 Sep 2006;**38**(9):623-642. Available from: https://pubmed.ncbi.nlm.nih.gov/16766237/

[32] Stramara L, Hernandez L, Bloom BT, Durham C. Development of parenteral nutrition-associated liver disease and other adverse effects in neonates receiving SMOFlipid or intralipid. Journal of Parenteral and Enteral Nutrition. Nov 2020;**44**(8):1530-1534. Available from: https://pubmed.ncbi.nlm.nih.gov/32027047/

[33] Blumenstein I. GLP-2 analogues as first specific treatment of intestinal failure. Visceral Medicine. 2019;**35**(5):320-323

[34] Moltu SJ, Bronsky J, Embleton N, Gerasimidis K, Indrio F, Köglmeier J, et al. Nutritional management of the critically ill neonate: A position paper of the ESPGHAN committee on nutrition. Journal of Pediatric Gastroenterology and Nutrition. 2021;**73**(2):274-289. DOI: 10.1097/MPG.0000000000003076

Chapter 4

Trends in Plasma Vitamin D Levels among Exclusively Breastfed Preterm Infants

Victor Ayodeji Ayeni, Tinuade Adetutu Ogunlesi, Iyabode Olabisi Florence Dedeke and Olatunbosun Oladipupo Olawale

Abstract

Exclusively breastfed preterm babies are dependent almost entirely on the available vitamin D content of breast milk for their metabolic and physiologic needs. The breast milk content of vitamin D correlates with the serum levels of vitamin D in the mother. This study investigates the trend in plasma vitamin D levels of preterm neonates who are exclusively breastfed between birth and 10 weeks of life. The proportion of mothers with low plasma vitamin D levels at birth was 41.7%, while it was 50% in the preterm babies. The plasma vitamin D levels in infants showed a strong positive correlation with maternal plasma levels at birth. By the 10th week postnatal age, the proportion of mothers with low plasma vitamin D had reduced slightly to 39.6%, but the proportion of babies with low plasma vitamin D had increased significantly to 81.3% while being fed exclusively on breast milk. It is, therefore, recommended that pregnant women should have vitamin D supplementation and that babies delivered preterm should have vitamin D supplementation.

Keywords: preterm infant, vitamin D, exclusive breastfeeding, Nigeria, pregnant women

1. Introduction

Sources of vitamin D in early infancy include transplacental transfer, breast milk, and cutaneous production through sunlight exposure. The maternal vitamin D status significantly influences the amount of vitamin D transported across the placenta during foetal development, consequently affecting the vitamin D reserves at birth [1, 2]. The vitamin D content in human milk typically ranges between 12 and 60 U/L and is generally insufficient to meet the physiologic needs of the growing infant [1]. After delivery, infants who are breastfed, therefore, depend primarily on cutaneous synthesis, which tends to be low due to limited sun exposure, to maintain adequate vitamin D levels. The half-life of 1,25-dihydroxyvitamin D is only 4 hours, so it does not reflect the vitamin D stores in the body [3]. On the other hand, the half-life of 25-hydroxyvitamin D is estimated to be approximately 2 to 3 weeks [4]. This suggests that 25-hydroxyvitamin D is both more reflective of stores in the body and also more likely to be related to an infant's postnatal nutrition when assayed after 9 weeks postnatal age rather than what the baby acquired *in utero.*

Current evidence does not affirm that the metabolism of vitamin D in preterm infants significantly differs from that in term infants, particularly with respect to the intestinal absorption of vitamin D, as well as its 25- and 1α-hydroxylation [5]. The vitamin D3 levels in human breast milk are low, and only minimal amounts of 25-hydroxyvitamin D are transferred from maternal circulation to breast milk [6]. Additionally, the vitamin D content of breast milk is correlated with the serum levels of vitamin D in the mother [7]. Furthermore, several studies have shown that the level of vitamin D in the newborn depends on the level of vitamin D in the mother while pregnant, with possible deleterious effects on the pregnancy outcome and growth of the newborn [8–11].

Preterm delivery constitutes about 12% of all births in Nigeria [12], and with the wide adherence to the tenets of the Baby Friendly Initiative (BFI), which prescribes exclusive breastfeeding, irrespective of the length of gestation of the infant, unless non-exclusive breastfeeding is medically indicated [13, 14], it is essential to examine the perinatal maternal vitamin D status, and the pattern of vitamin D among Nigerian preterm infants, who are exclusively breastfed. According to the recommendations provided by the World Health Organisation (WHO) for the optimal feeding of low-birth-weight infants, the evidence for feeding babies exclusively on breastmilk is strong for low- and middle-income countries. However, the evidence supporting supplementation with substances other than breast milk (including vitamin D) is weak [15]. In contrast, some studies in Caucasian and Asian countries [16–18] suggest that the supplementation with vitamin D is beneficial in preterm and low-birth-weight babies. The study, therefore, aims to determine the trend in mean plasma levels of vitamin D from birth to 10 weeks postnatal age in a Nigerian population of exclusively breastfed preterm infants while comparing these with plasma levels in their corresponding mothers at birth and at 10 weeks postnatal age.

2. Methods

2.1 Study design

This was a hospital-based panel study that took place in three hospitals within Ogun State, southwest Nigeria. The study sites were Olabisi Onabanjo University Teaching Hospital, Sagamu, Federal Medical Centre, Abeokuta, and Sacred Heart Hospital, Abeokuta, all in Ogun State. All three hospitals were designated centres for specialised obstetric and paediatric care.

2.2 Study population, sampling, and eligibility criteria

The study subjects included singleton preterm neonates born before an estimated gestational age (EGA) of 37 completed weeks and aged between 0 and 24 hours in any of the study sites, as well as their paired mothers. The exclusion criteria included milk feeding prior to presentation at the study sites, maternal diabetes, maternal prolonged use of anticonvulsant drugs, tocolytic agents and magnesium sulphate in pregnancy and perinatally, presence of gross malformations of the digestive tract and central nervous system and any other severe illness, which precluded oral feeding in the infant. The studied infants were the number of infants who were eligible for follow-up for vitamin D levels at 10 weeks, from a larger study. The rest of the recruited baby in the larger study had died (19%), were erroneously fed artificial milk (6.6%), were lost to follow-up (19%) or were given medications that could alter vitamin D metabolism (15.7%), by the time of follow-up at 10 weeks postnatal age. This is shown in **Figure 1**. The mothers and their babies were consecutively recruited at the Postnatal Ward in the Maternity Unit of each of the hospitals (for in-born babies), as well as the Neonatal Unit (for out-born babies).

2.3 Data collection process

Data were collected between April 2018 and February 2020. A research proforma in the form of a structured questionnaire was used for the study. The documented data included maternal age, maternal parity, last confinement, mode of feeding following birth, history of medications used during pregnancy, and perinatally, age and sex of the baby. The body weight, body length, and occipitofrontal circumference (OFC) of the babies were taken at each contact. The body weight was measured to the nearest 10 g, while the recumbent body length and occipitofrontal circumference were measured to the nearest 0.1 cm [19]. The EGA by Ballard Scoring was determined for each neonate, using the New Ballard Scoring system [20].

Contacts were made with the subjects within the first 24 hours of life and at the 10th week of postnatal age. All recruited infants received 0.3 ml/day of multivitamin drops, which contained 200 IU of ergocalciferol, in accordance with the unit protocols at the study sites and as ethically recommended. The parents were counselled on exclusive breastfeeding, using the method prescribed by the managing physicians (either direct suckling only or direct suckling with supplemental expressed breast milk).

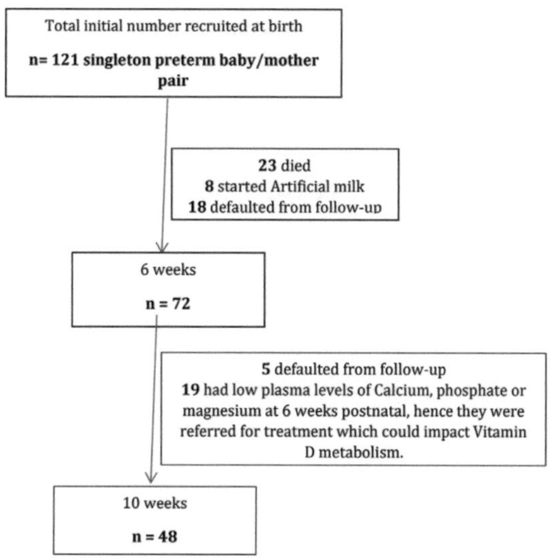

Figure 1.
Flow chart of selected babies.

2.4 Blood sample collection, storage, and analysis

At both contacts, 2 millilitres of venous blood samples were taken from each mother and infant for the laboratory assay of plasma vitamin D. The blood sample was promptly taken to the laboratory and was centrifuged at 2000–3000 g for 15 minutes, to separate the plasma from the cells, within 1 hour of sample collection [21]. The plasma was then decanted into a clean serum bottle and transported/stored at a temperature of −20°C. The assay was performed using a solid phase 25-OH vitamin D Total ELISA (Enzyme-Linked Immunosorbent Assay) Kit manufactured by Demeditec Diagnostics®, GmbH, Germany. The reference range for normal plasma levels of 25-OH vitamin D was 30–100 ng/ml.

2.5 Data management

The data were analysed, using the Statistical Package for the Social Sciences (SPSS) 26.0 software (IBM Corp). Analyses were done using descriptive and inferential statistics. Mean values of continuous variables were compared using the *Student's t-test* or Analysis of variance *(ANOVA).* Proportions of continuous variables were compared using the *Chi-Square* test. Correlation analysis (*Pearson's r or Spearman's rho*) was used to describe relationships between continuous variables. Statistical significance was determined using p-values less than 0.05.

2.6 Ethical considerations

Ethical approval was obtained from the Health Research Ethics Committees of Olabisi Onabanjo University Teaching Hospital, Sagamu (OOUTH/HREC/119/2017); Federal Medical Centre, Abeokuta (FMCA/47/HREC/10/2017); and Sacred Heart Hospital, Abeokuta (SHH/EC/EA/003/08/17). The mothers/−caregivers of all eligible participants were given detailed information about the study. Written informed consent was obtained from the mothers/caregivers present at the point of enrolment into the study.

3. Results

A total of 48 mother-preterm infant pairs recruited were followed up for 10 weeks. The babies' birth weights ranged from 0.68 to 3.31 kg, with a mean of 1.997 ± 0.571 kg. The mean length at birth was 43.0 ± 4.1 cm, with a range of 32.9–51.0 cm. The occipitofrontal circumference at birth ranged from 22.5 to 35.0 cm, with a mean of 30.3 ± 3.0 cm. The EGA ranged from 26 to 36 weeks, with a mean of 33.3 ± 2.3 weeks and a median of 34 weeks. There were slightly more males, 25/48 (52.1%). The ages of the mothers ranged from 21 to 45 years, with a mean of 31.2 ± 5.7 years. Parity at the time of recruitment ranged from one to six (1 to 6). Mothers whose last confinement fell within 2–10 years had the highest frequency of 27 (56%), and primiparous mothers were 14 (29.2%).

3.1 Plasma vitamin D levels at birth

The mean plasma vitamin D level in the mothers was 33.26 ± 11.79 ng/mL (range = 2.69–78.20 ng/mL), and hypovitaminosis D was recorded in 20/48 (41.7%)

of the mothers (**Figure 1**). The mean plasma vitamin D level at birth in the babies was 30.95 ± 11.11 ng/mL, with a range of 8.70–59.96 ng/mL. Twenty-four (50%) babies had low levels of vitamin D (**Figure 2**). There was a moderate positive correlation between maternal plasma vitamin D levels at birth and their corresponding neonatal substrate levels at birth ($r = 0.612; p < 0.001$).

Most of the infants of mothers who had normal plasma vitamin D levels at birth also had normal plasma vitamin D, while most of the infants of mothers who had low plasma vitamin D levels at birth also had low plasma vitamin D ($\chi^2 = 16.800; p < 0.001$).

3.2 Plasma vitamin D levels at 10 weeks

At 10 weeks, the mean plasma vitamin D in the mothers was 32.72 ± 8.27 ng/mL, with a range of 17.80–58.73 ng/mL. Plasma vitamin D levels were low in 19/48 (39.6%) of the mothers (**Figure 3**). The mean plasma vitamin D in the infants at 10 weeks age was 23.56 ± 8.64 ng/mL with a range of 3.40–47.13 ng/mL. Plasma vitamin D levels were low in 39/48 (81.3%) babies (**Figure 3**). There was no significant relationship between the categories of plasma vitamin D in the infant at 10 weeks when compared with the category of corresponding maternal plasma vitamin D at 10 weeks ($\chi^2 = 0.109$; p = 0.741).

3.3 Comparison of demographic characteristics of the mothers and babies in relation to vitamin D levels

Table 1 shows the distribution of maternal vitamin D levels in mothers at birth in relation to their educational level and ages, while **Table 2** shows the distribution at 10 weeks. The difference was not statistically significant in the categories. **Table 3** shows the babies' plasma vitamin D levels in relation to the babies' sex at birth and at 10 weeks. The sex had no significant association with the category of vitamin D levels both at birth and at 10 weeks postnatal ages.

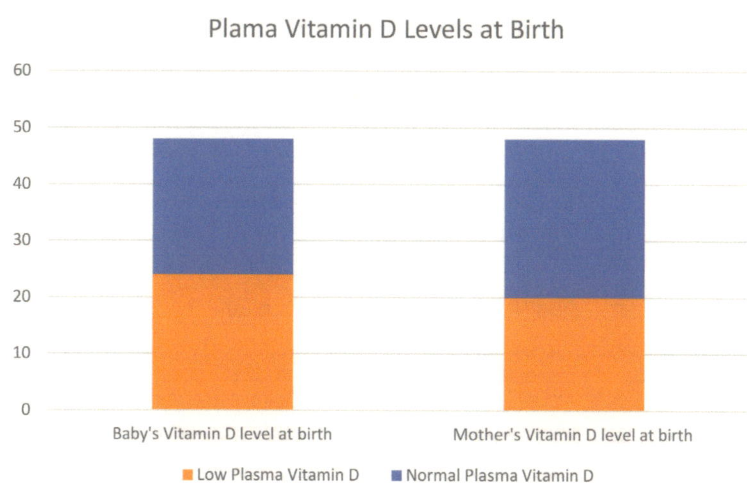

Figure 2.
Plasma vitamin D levels in the babies and mothers at birth.

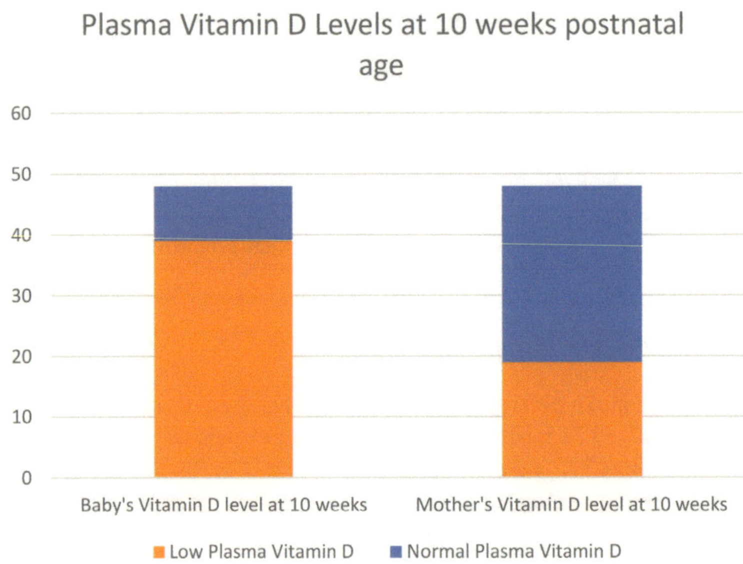

Figure 3.
Plasma vitamin D levels in the babies and mothers at 10 weeks postnatal age.

Characteristic	Low maternal vitamin D (%)	Normal maternal vitamin D (%)	Chi-Square	P-value
Educational Level			1.317	0.251
Primary & Secondary	6 (31.6)	13 (68.4)		
Post-Secondary	14 (48.3)	15 (51.7)		
Maternal Age			0.148	0.701
20–35 years	14 (40.0)	21 (60.0)		
> 35 years	6 (46.2)	7 (53.8)		

Table 1.
Plasma vitamin D categories in the mothers at birth in relation to maternal sociodemographic characteristics.

Characteristic	Low maternal vitamin D (%)	Normal maternal vitamin D (%)	Chi-Square	P-value
Educational Level			0.084	0.772
Primary & Secondary	8 (42.1)	11 (57.9)		
Post-Secondary	11 (37.9)	18 (62.1)		
Maternal Age			0.322	0.571
20–35 years	13 (37.1)	22 (62.9)		
> 35 years	6 (46.2)	7 (53.8)		

Table 2.
Plasma vitamin D categories in the mothers at 10 weeks in relation to maternal sociodemographic characteristics.

Characteristic	Low vitamin D (%)	Normal vitamin D (%)	Chi-Square	P-value
At birth				
Female	10 (43.5)	13 (56.5)	0.751	0.386
Male	14 (56.0)	11 (44.0)		
At 10 weeks				
Female	18 (78.3)	5 (21.7)	0.259	0.611
Male	21 (84.0)	4 (16.0)		

Table 3.
Plasma vitamin D categories in the babies at birth and at 10 weeks in relation to the sex of the babies.

Variables	Pearson coefficient (r)	p-value
Maternal vitamin D at birth and Maternal vitamin D at 10 weeks	0.245	0.094
Baby's vitamin D at birth and Baby's vitamin D at 10 weeks	0.279	0.054
Maternal vitamin D at 10 weeks and Baby's vitamin D at 10 weeks	−0.070	0.636

Table 4.
Correlations between plasma vitamin D levels at birth and 10 weeks among infants and their mothers.

3.4 Comparison of mean plasma vitamin D levels at birth and at 10 weeks

Table 4 shows weakly positive and insignificant correlations between maternal plasma vitamin D levels at birth and at 10 weeks, as well as between the babies' plasma vitamin D levels at birth and at 10 weeks. Similarly, the correlation between plasma vitamin D levels in infants and mothers at 10 weeks was negative, weak, and insignificant. There was no significant relationship between the categories of plasma vitamin D in the infant at 10 weeks when compared with the category of corresponding maternal plasma vitamin D at birth (χ^2 = 0.031; p = 0.854). Similarly, the relationship between categories of plasma vitamin D in the babies at birth and at 10 weeks was not significant (χ^2 = 0.137; p = 0.712).

4. Discussion

Fifty percent of the babies in the present study had low plasma vitamin D at birth. The finding on neonatal plasma vitamin D in the present study is also similar to that reported earlier by Terek et al. in Turkey [22], in which about half of the babies had low vitamin D levels. However, a study in India [23] found a vitamin D deficiency prevalence of 92% in preterm neonates, using the cutoff of 30 ng/dL used in this study. The Indian study did not include maternal vitamin D levels, which have been shown to have a direct correlation with the baby's vitamin D levels [11, 24]. Hence it would be difficult to explain the marked variation without also considering the maternal values.

The mean neonatal plasma vitamin D at birth was significantly lower than the mean maternal plasma levels of vitamin D in the present study. The relative disparity in the levels of low vitamin D in the neonates, accords with the findings in an

Australian study by Panda et al. [25], This may be simply related to the normal physiology in foetal life requiring a relatively low parathormone and a low 1,25-dihydroxyvitamin D for optimal bone mineralisation *in utero* [5, 26]. On the other hand, the mean neonatal plasma vitamin D levels had a direct positive correlation with the maternal levels, as previously established in previous studies [11, 24].

The low neonatal plasma vitamin D levels found in this study are a direct reflection of the maternal vitamin D levels, and this accords with previous reports [1, 2, 8, 25, 27]. Vitamin D deficiency is known to be common in pregnant women and breastfed infants, despite the use of vitamin supplementation in pregnant women [28], with negative implications for both pregnancy outcomes and infant growth and development [29, 30].

The present study showed that there was no correlation between plasma vitamin D at 10 weeks and plasma vitamin D at birth. This is to be expected because the half-life of plasma 25-hydroxyvitamin D is only 3 weeks [4], so the plasma vitamin D levels at 10 weeks could be adjudged to be dependent on the available dietary sources, which is breast milk in this cohort of babies. It should be noted that the babies in this study were given a supplement of daily 200 IU of vitamin D, according to the standard protocols in the hospitals at the time of the study, but this did not significantly improve the vitamin D levels. Conversely, the proportion of babies with low plasma vitamin D increased to four-fifths at 10 weeks postnatal age, from only half at birth, despite supplementation with a daily dose of 200 IU of vitamin D! This suggests that not only is there the need for supplementation in the Nigerian population studied, but also that the optimal doses should be more than 200 IU. This aligns with the doses of 400 IU or higher for vitamin D supplementation in preterm neonates highlighted in previous studies on neonates in Asia, Europe, North America, and Australia/New Zealand [16–18]. Different studies, specifically in preterm neonates, have reported varying recommendations. Some studies carried out in Republic of Ireland and Turkey [31, 32] suggest that supplementing with 400 IU of vitamin D daily achieved sufficient levels of 25 hydroxyvitamin D in infants. On the other hand, some trials conducted in India [16, 33] reported that doses of 1000 IU daily of oral vitamin D are more effective to achieve optimal levels.

Furthermore, it is important to pay attention to the reducing levels of vitamin D in preterm neonates if they are given only breastmilk without oral vitamin D supplementation at optimal quantities. Supplementation with vitamin D in deficient infants has been known to reduce the risk of respiratory infections and autoimmune diseases [34], protect against nutritional rickets [17], and improve the growth of preterm neonates [18]. These effects could not be investigated in this cohort of preterm neonates because of the small sample size and early follow-up period. Nonetheless, in the face of WHO recommendations for low- and middle-income countries about the need for supplementation or not for exclusively breastfed preterm infants [15], the findings from this study are a wakeup call for more high-powered studies to investigate the long-term consequences of non-supplementation of breastmilk in preterm babies. The study also highlights the need to conduct trials to determine the optimal dosing regimen of enteral supplemental vitamin D to maintain adequate plasma levels of vitamin D in babies who are delivered preterm in the population studied. The limitations of the present study include its small sample size and short follow-up duration.

5. Conclusion and recommendations

Fifty percent of the singleton preterm babies had low plasma levels of vitamin D at birth. There were strongly positive correlations between maternal and neonatal plasma vitamin D levels at birth. The proportion of babies with low vitamin D levels increased to 81.3% by 10 weeks while on exclusive breastfeeding and supplementation with 200 IU of vitamin D daily. However, the proportion of mothers with low vitamin D reduced slightly, meaning that the worsening vitamin D levels in the babies were due to inadequate quantities from the breastmilk source. Hence, routine supplementation of vitamin D and preterm infants who are exclusively breastfed is recommended at doses greater than 200 IU per day. Further studies are required to determine optimal quantities of vitamin D to give as a supplement for pregnant women and preterm neonates in the population studied.

Acknowledgements

We thank Dr. Idayat Oguntade, Dr. Oluwafemi Oshin and Dr. James Eniola for their help with blood sample collection at odd times during the period of the study. We also appreciate Drs. Opeyemi Kuponiyi, Olubunmi Oba-Daini, Udoka Adeniyi, Adebimpe Adesanya, Ayopo Atunwa, Fatimat Olorunjuwon, and Tolulope Asare for their help in the sample selection process.

Conflict of interest

The authors declare no conflict of interest.

List of abbreviations

BFI	baby friendly initiative
EGA	estimated gestational age
ELISA	enzyme-linked immunosorbent assay
OFC	occipitofrontal circumference
SPSS	statistical package for the social sciences
WHO	world health organisation

Author details

Victor Ayodeji Ayeni[1*], Tinuade Adetutu Ogunlesi[2], Iyabode Olabisi Florence Dedeke[3] and Olatunbosun Oladipupo Olawale[4]

1 Department of Paediatrics, Babcock University, Ilishan-Remo, Nigeria

2 Department of Paediatrics, Olabisi Onabanjo University, Ago-Iwoye, Nigeria

3 Department of Paediatrics, Federal Medical Centre, Abeokuta, Nigeria

4 Department of Chemical Pathology, Olabisi Onabanjo University, Ago-Iwoye, Nigeria

*Address all correspondence to: tioluwa@hotmail.com

References

[1] Hatun S, Ozkan B, Orbak Z, Doneray H, Cizmecioglu F, Toprak D, et al. Vitamin D deficiency in early infancy. The Journal of Nutrition. 2005;**135**(2):279-282

[2] Wagner CL, Greer FR. Prevention of rickets and vitamin D deficiency in infants, children, and adolescents. Pediatrics. 2008;**122**(5):1142-1152

[3] Misra M, Pacaud D, Petryk A, Collett-Solberg PF, Kappy M. Vitamin D deficiency in children and its management: Review of current knowledge and recommendations. Pediatrics. 2008;**122**(2):398-417

[4] Merewood A, Mehta SD, Grossman X, Chen TC, Mathieu J, Holick MF, et al. Vitamin D status among 4-month-old infants in New England. Journal of Human Lactation [Internet]. 2012;**28**(2):159-166. DOI: 10.1177/0890334411434802

[5] Mimouni FB, Mandel D, Lubetzky R, Senterre T. Calcium, phosphorus, magnesium and vitamin D requirements of the preterm infant. In: Koletzko B, Poindexter B, Uauy R, editors. Nutritional Care of Preterm Infants: Scientific Basis and Practical Guidelines. World Review of Nutrition and Dietetics [Internet]. Basel: Karger; 2014. pp. 140-151. Available from: https://www.karger.com/Article/FullText/358463

[6] Bae YJ, Kratzsch J. Vitamin D and calcium in the human breast milk. Best Practice & Research Clinical Endocrinology & Metabolism. 2018;**32**(1):39-45

[7] Butte NF, Garza C, Johnson CA, Smith EOB, Nichols BL. Longitudinal changes in milk composition of mothers delivering preterm and term infants. Early Human Development. 1984;**9**(2):153-162

[8] Jamali Z, Ghorbani F, Shafie'ei M, Tolooefar F, Maleki E. Risk factors associated with vitamin D deficiency in preterm neonates: A single-center step-wise regression analysis. BMC Pediatrics. 2023;**23**(1)

[9] Pérez-López FR, Pilz S, Chedraui P. Vitamin D supplementation during pregnancy: An overview. Current Opinion in Obstetrics & Gynecology. 2020;**32**(5):316-321

[10] Wei SQ. Vitamin D and pregnancy outcomes. Current Opinion in Obstetrics & Gynecology [Internet]. 2014;**26**(6):438-447. Available from: https://pubmed.ncbi.nlm.nih.gov/25310531/

[11] Ayeni VA, Ogunlesi TA, IOF D, Olawale OO, Olanrewaju DM. Plasma vitamin D levels among Nigerian mothers and their preterm infants. West African Journal of Medicine [Internet]. 2024;**41**(5):555-561. Available from: https://pubmed.ncbi.nlm.nih.gov/39207936/

[12] Mokuolu OA, Suleiman BM, Adesiyun OO, Adeniyi A. Prevalence and determinants of pre-term deliveries in the University of Ilorin Teaching Hospital, Ilorin, Nigeria. Pediatric Reports. 2010;**2**(1):11-14

[13] WHO. Global strategy for infant and young child feeding. In: Global Strategy for Infant and Young Child Feeding. Geneva: World Health Organization; 2003. pp. 7-8

[14] WHO. Recommendations. In: Guidelines on Optimal Feeding of Low

Birth- Weight Infants in Low-and Middle-Income Countries. Geneva: World Health Organization; 2011. pp. 16-45

[15] WHO recommendations for care of the preterm or low-birth-weight infant [Internet]. Available from: https://www.who.int/publications/i/item/9789240058262 [Accessed: April 15, 2024]

[16] Mathur NB, Saini A, Mishra TK. Assessment of adequacy of supplementation of vitamin D in very low birth weight preterm neonates: A randomized controlled trial. Journal of Tropical Pediatrics. 2016;**62**(6):429-435

[17] Zittermann A, Pilz S, Berthold HK. Serum 25-hydroxyvitamin D response to vitamin D supplementation in infants: A systematic review and meta-analysis of clinical intervention trials. European Journal of Nutrition [Internet]. 2020;**59**(1):359-369. Available from: https://link.springer.com/article/10.1007/s00394-019-01912-x

[18] Kumar M, Shaikh S, Sinha B, Prakash Upadhyay R, Choudhary TS, Rongsen Chandola T, et al. Enteral vitamin D supplementation in preterm or low birth weight infants: A systematic review and meta-analysis. Pediatrics [Internet]. 2022;**150**(S1):e2022057092K. Available from: https://doi.org/2022057092K

[19] Centres for Disease Control and Prevention. Anthropometry procedures manual. In: National Health and Nutrition Examination Survey (NHANES) [Internet]. Hyattsville: U.S. Department of Health and Human Services, Centers for Disease Control and Prevention; 2007. pp. 30-56. Available from: http://www.cdc.gov/nchs/data/nhanes/nhanes_07_08/manual_an.pdf

[20] Ballard JL, Khoury JC, Wedig K, Wang L, Eilers-Walsman BL, Lipp R. New Ballard score, expanded to include extremely premature infants. The Journal of Pediatrics. 1991;**119**(3):417-423

[21] WHO. Analyte stability in sample matrix. In: Use of Anticoagulants in Diagnostic Laboratory Investigations. Geneva: World Health Organization; 2002. p. 10

[22] Terek D, Ozcan G, Ergin F, Koroglu OA, Yalz M, Akisu M, et al. Vitamin D deficiency in premature infants and its effects on neonatal prognosis. The Journal of Pediatric Research. 2018;**5**(1):37-40

[23] Dadwal M, Narayan R. A study of pattern of vitamin D deficiency in preterm and term newborns at rural teaching hospital, Haryana, India. Sri Lanka Journal of Child Health. 2020;**49**(3):251-255

[24] Ayeni VA. A narrative review of calcium, phosphate, magnesium and vitamin D metabolism in breastfed preterm babies. Nigerian Journal of Paediatrics. 2024;**51**(2):55-64

[25] Panda M, McIntosh J, Chaudhari T, Kent AL. Do maternal vitamin D levels influence vitamin D levels in preterm neonates? International Journal of Pediatrics (United Kingdom). 2019;**2019**(1):8613414

[26] Land C, Schoenau E. Fetal and postnatal bone development: Reviewing the role of mechanical stimuli and nutrition. Best Practice and Research in Clinical Endocrinology and Metabolism. 2008;**22**(1):107-118

[27] Kassai MS, Cafeo FR, Affonso-Kaufman FA, Suano-souza FI. Vitamin D plasma concentrations in pregnant women and their preterm newborns. BMC Pregnancy Childbirth. 2018;**18**:412

[28] Mulligan ML, Felton SK, Riek AE, Bernal-Mizrachi C. Implications of vitamin D deficiency in pregnancy and lactation. American Journal of Obstetrics and Gynecology. 2010;**202**(5):429.e1-429.e9

[29] Zhang H, Wang S, Tuo L, Zhai Q, Cui J, Chen D, et al. Relationship between maternal vitamin D levels and adverse outcomes. Nutrients [Internet]. 2022;**14**(20):4230. Available from: https://pubmed.ncbi.nlm.nih.gov/36296914/ [Accessed: October 14, 2023]

[30] von Websky K, Hasan AA, Reichetzeder C, Tsuprykov O, Hocher B. Impact of vitamin D on pregnancy-related disorders and on offspring outcome. Journal of Steroid Biochemistry and Molecular Biology. 2018;**180**:51-64

[31] McCarthy RA, McKenna MJ, Oyefeso O, Uduma O, Murray BF, Brady JJ, et al. Vitamin D nutritional status in preterm infants and response to supplementation. British Journal of Nutrition. 2013;**110**(1):156-163

[32] Sarldemir H, Surmeli Onay O, Aydemir O, Tekin AN. Questioning the adequacy of standardized vitamin D supplementation protocol in very low birth weight infants: A prospective cohort study. Journal of Pediatric Endocrinology and Metabolism [Internet]. 2021;**34**(12):1515-1523. DOI: 10.1515/jpem-2021-0390/html

[33] Tergestina M, Rebekah G, Job V, Simon A, Thomas N. A randomized double-blind controlled trial comparing two regimens of vitamin D supplementation in preterm neonates. Journal of Perinatology. 2016;**36**(9):763-767

[34] Mansur JL, Oliveri B, Giacoia E, Fusaro D, Costanzo PR. Vitamin D: Before, during and after pregnancy: Effect on neonates and children. Nutrients. 2022;**14**(9):1900

Chapter 5

Neonatal Endocrinology

Dragan Katanić

Abstract

Endocrine processes are fundamental and evolutionary older than neural system. Neonatal endocrinology covers perinatal period, auxology, thyroid function, calcium and bone metabolism, glucose homeostasis, adrenal gland disorders, sex differentiation, water balance, endocrine disruptors, and syndromatology. All this orchestra in harmony, with hypothalamus like conductor and pituitary like the first violin, is needed for normal development, and its disorder sometimes may explain reasons for critically ill newborns or emergency. Transition from fetal life, maternal endocrine diseases, and placental hormones even more complicate comprehension. Clinical signs and assessment, investigations, and treatment are discussed, offering the basic knowledge for young endocrinologists and pediatricians.

Keywords: endocrinology, newborn, auxology, thyroid, calcium metabolism, neonatal diabetes, adrenal axis, sex differentiation

1. Introduction

Endocrine pathology in the neonatal age is not common, but it can be fatal in course, urging for quick decisions, missing cooperation from the little patient, could leave consequences for life and demand lifelong treatment. Emergencies include hypoglycemia, salt losing syndrome (congenital adrenal hyperplasia), neonatal diabetes, and hyperthyroidism. Screening for congenital hypothyroidism is never complete and could be false negative, and it is necessary to recognize the clinical pattern in time, in order to prevent severe mental and growth retardation. Syndromatology in this period has also important role, and interpretation of hormonal profile is age specific, even more complex in infants born prematurely. The chapter describes signs and symptoms of endocrine disorders and gives practical clinical guidance for timely recognition and management of neonatal endocrine pathology.

2. Fetal endocrinology

In the formation of the endocrine glands, all germ layers are involved—ectoderm (neurohypophysis, C-cells of the parathyroid glands, and adrenal medulla), endoderm (adenohypophysis, thyroid gland, parathyroid glands, and pancreas), and mesoderm (adrenal cortex and gonads). Their vascularization is ample because hormones are secreted directly into the blood, and not through the excretory duct. The endocrine axes of the fetus are established in the middle of gestation.

Three endocrine organs descend during embryonic development—the neurohypophysis, the thyroid gland, and the testicles. Due to the complicated development, congenital anomalies often occur on them (ectopia of the neurohypophysis, Rathke cyst, medial cyst of the neck due to remnant of thyroglossal duct, cryptorchidism).

Parathyroid glands are formed from the pharyngeal pouches. Their first neighbor is thymus, and lesions of the parathyroid glands are often associated with a decline in cellular immunity and mycoses (DiGeorge syndrome).

3. Placenta

The placenta is at the same time a link and a barrier, as well as a place of hormone production. Human choriogonadotropin (hCG) stimulates the thyroid gland of the mother (which should work for two), and the high level of this hormone favors hyperemesis gravidarum and the formation of neonatal ovarian cysts. Placental lactogen (human chorionic somatomammotropin) with its hyperglycemic effect provides energy to the fetus, but in genetically predisposed pregnant women it favors gestational diabetes.

Glucose easily passes through the placenta, and maternal hyperglycemia (diabetes) leads to hyperplasia of fetal beta-cells, fetal macrosomia, and large newborns because, in utero, the action of the insulin-like family (insulin-like growth factors) is important for growth [1, 2].

Calcium easily crosses the placenta to the fetus, and the parathyroid glands of the newborn might therefore be dormant for the first few days (transient neonatal hypocalcemia).

Iodides easily pass placenta as a nutrient or as a diagnostic and therapeutic agent (that is why scintigraphy and treatment of hyperthyroidism with radioactive iodine are contraindicated in pregnancy). Thyrostatics do the same (resulting in transient hypothyroidism of the newborn) and also thyroid stimulating immunoglobuline (TSI) belonging to the tiny IgG class, leading to transient hyperthyroidism of the newborn.

4. Peripartum endocrinology

4.1 Hormonal mechanisms of initiation of labor

The initiation of labor originates from the fetus (due to the lack of space and energy for further growth). After 9 months spent in a safe shelter, on delivery the newborns find themselves in a completely new environment. The ambient temperature drops from 37°C (intrauterine) to lower in the delivery room, the influx of energy (glucose) is no longer continuous, but intermittent (meals) and different (milk lipids). Cutting of the umbilicus, rapid expansion of the lungs, oxygenation, prostaglandins, and torsion of ductus arteriosus lead to the adaptation of the pulmonary and cardiovascular systems.

The lower extremities at birth are very short (the ratio of the upper to the lower segment is 1.7, around the age of 11 it is 1, and after puberty it is 0.9). The head makes up 1/4 of the body at birth and about 1/6 of the body length at adulthood.

4.2 Stress hormone response during childbirth (functional trauma)

Childbirth, especially difficult one, is a great stress, and all stress hormones rise sharply:

- Adrenocorticotropic hormone (ACTH) and cortisol provide glucose (by gluconeogenesis), the body's principal energy source, and prevent massive bleeding during childbirth. However, a high concentration of cortisol could favor microthromboses due to its procoagulant effect, especially in the newborn with polycythemia;
- Prolactin (PRL) has a stimulating effect on the glomerulose zone and, by retaining sodium, increases blood pressure (and improves tissue perfusion); also neutralizes the negative impact of hypercortisolemia on cellular immunity (immuno-modulator);
- Adrenaline, by glycogenolysis, also provides glucose (the main fuel) and leads to tachycardia;
- Norepinephrine is associated with greater stress intensity and causes bradycardia, which requires the use of atropine;
- Antidiuretic hormone (ADH) by retaining water (which has a large heat capacity) prevents overheating of muscles;
- Endorphins have an analgesic effect.

4.3 Anatomical injuries of the endocrine glands (physical trauma)

The adrenal glands are most often exposed to injuries due to their size and location. In the newborn, they are relatively large, spongy, and highly vascularized, so the pressure of the obstetrician's hands on the rib arches of the mother (where the projection of the glands is) easily leads to intraadrenal hemorrhage.

Anatomical injuries of the thyroid gland during delivery are extremely rare and occur only with large congenital goiter, due to dyshormogenesis and a consecutive increase in fetal TSH from the midgestation.

Torsion or lesion of the testicles can occur during a difficult or rapid birth, due to their position.

True intrapartum injuries of the parathyroid glands are rare. If, in the context of a difficult birth, one of them is injured, the others will compensatory take over its function, which is an evolutionary defense against hypocalcemia, since calcium, in addition to osteosynthesis, is essential for adequate blood coagulation and neuromuscular activity.

Injuries of the hypothalamic-pituitary complex occur within the presentatio pelvina, when hyperextension of the head of the newborn occurs during expulsion, or in the case of trauma (including abuse).

5. Neonatal auxology

5.1 Small for gestational age (SGA)

Endocrinological criteria for assessing the growth of the fetus and newborn are based on body weight and body length. Data obtained by fetal ultrasound are compared to standard growth curves for races and ethnicities [3, 4]. Growth and/or weight below −2 SD (below the tenth percentile) indicates a newborn small gestational age (SGA). They are also called "small for date." By following up these children, it has been observed that most of them reach the physical development of their peers by the age of 6 months or 2 years, and no later than their fourth birthday (catch up growth). For SGA children who fail to do so and do not have any other pathological condition (e.g., hypothyroidism and celiac disease), the administration of growth hormone is indicated, without prior determination of the pituitary capacity for growth hormone by dynamic (stimulating) tests. Thus, the criterion for the introduction of growth hormone is auxological, not laboratory. This group of children may have health problems during childhood (logoretardation, attention deficit disorder) and in adulthood (short stature, osteoporosis, metabolic syndrome, and lower IQ). Growth hormone shows a beneficial preventive effect on all of the above conditions. In mnemonics for children born small for gestational age, the central mnemonic place is occupied by the number 10:

- 10th percentile (or less) of length and/or weight at birth by definition
- 10% of newborns are born small for gestational age
- 10% of them do not catch up height by their 4th birthday
- 10% will develop metabolic syndrome in their lifetime
- 10 cm will be lower than their genetic potential (midparental height).

Newborns small for gestational age are also part of the of Silver-Russell, de Morsier (septo-optic dysplasia), Turner and Prader-Willi-Labhart syndrome.

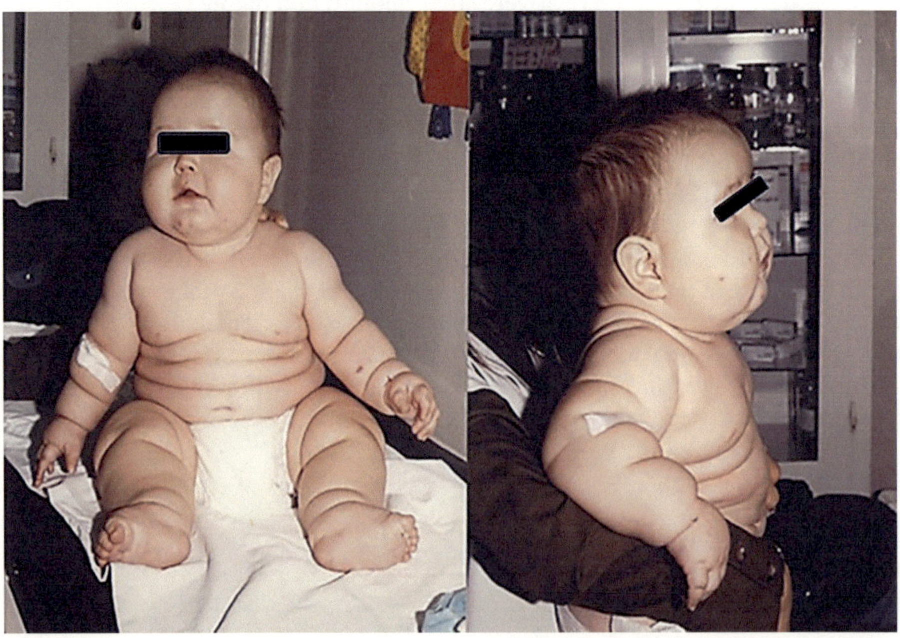

Figure 1.
Sotos syndrome.

5.2 Large for gestational age (LGA)

The background of these conditions is fetal hyperinsulinemia, since in fetal life the insulin family is a growth factor. They are present within the syndrome of Beckwith-Wiedemann,[1] Sotos[2] (**Figure 1**), Perlman, Simpson-Golabi-Behmel ("Bulldog"), in the child of a pregnant woman with diabetes, etc.

It is important to mention that children with congenital hypothyroidism are also born with a bigger weight (and average length), due to fluid retention.

6. Disorders of thyroid function

After childbirth, due to the lower temperature of the environment, moist skin of the newborn, and a limited amount of adipose tissue, the newborn is prone to hypothermia. The first defense against cooling is the hypothalamic-pituitary-thyroid axis and the sudden spike in thyroid-stimulating hormone (TSH) and triiodothyronine (T3), which, by stimulating the activity of the mitochondria of the brown adipose tissue surrounding adrenals, rapidly heat the body. Thus, physiological hyperthyrotropinemia (elevated TSH) is seen in the first few days, directly proportional to the difference in temperature in utero and intra muros. Therefore, blood for screening for TSH-based congenital hypothyroidism is never taken for the first 2 days after birth, nor from the umbilical cord.

Newborns (5–30 days of life) and infants have higher levels of thyroid binding globulin (TBG) and different acceptable hormone range [5] than adults (**Table 1**).

6.1 Congenital hypothyroidism

Permanent congenital hypothyroidism occurs due to an anatomical defect (aplasia or ectopia of the gland) or a lack of enzymes (dyshormogenesis—then, due to high TSH, goiter is already present at birth). Transient congenital hypothyroidism may be the result of iodine deficiency (in endemic areas), transplacental crossing of blocking antibodies or thyrostatic agents, and prematurity.

The clinical picture of a child with congenital hypothyroidism (**Figure 2**) is the result of the absence of diuretic, thermogenic, neurotropic, cardiotropic, and favorable effect of thyrohormones on growth and metabolism.

Hormone	Normal range
TSH (mU/L)	1–10
T4 (nmol/L)	75–220
T3 (nmol/L)	1.3–4.5
fT4 (pmol/L)	11–23
fT3 (pmol/L)	3–7

Table 1.
Normal values of thyroid hormones in the neonatal period.

[1] "Has everything big (organomegaly), only the sugar is small."
[2] "A big kid who later cannot ride a bicycle (clumsy) and has often a sella facing backwards."

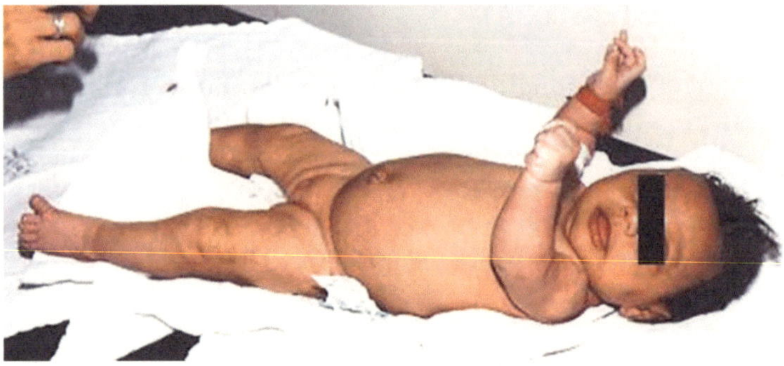

Figure 2.
Child with cogenital hypothyroidism.

Due to the lack of thyroid hormones, fluid retention occurs, which is manifested by generalized swelling (anasarca) and increased birth weight, swelling of the eyelids (narrowed palpebral fissure), congestion of the nasal mucosa, lingual lymphedema (constant protrusion of the tongue), swelling of the vocal cords (low-tonality crying, laryngeal stridor), and effusion into the serous cavities. The length of a child with congenital hypothyroidism is usually normal at birth. Due to reduced thermogenesis, hypothermia occurs, which vitally threatens the newborn.

Since, postnatally, thyroid hormones are important for the maturation (arborization, myelinization, and synaptogenesis) of the central nervous system, their deficiency in this critical period (the first 2 weeks and until the end of the third month of life) irreversibly damages it and leaves tragic consequences on neurocognitive development (cretinism).

In the absence of thyroid hormones, which act positively inotropic, positively chronotropic, positively dromotropic, and negatively batmotropic, the ECG shows microvoltage and sinus bradycardia.

Slower metabolism leads to lethargy and hypotonia (often accompanied by hernias), attenuated reflexes, delayed meconium evacuation and constipation, anemia, hyperbilirubinemia, hypercholesterolemia, dry skin, and delayed ossification (the small fontanel at birth has a diameter of more than 0.5 cm, the nose is saddle due to insufficiency of osteogenesis, the ossification center of the distal epiphysis of the femur is often missing, and ultrasonography usually finds immature hip architecture).

Didactically, it can be said that a newborn with congenital hypothyroidism sleeps a lot, does not require frequent changing diapers (constipation), sucks poorly and rarely cries. It is "a large, lemon-yellow, limp newborn, which thrives poorly and is easy to care for."

Replacement therapy is levothyroxine 10–15 mcg/kg/day orally (introduced gradually within few days to avoid cardiac strain). An attempt to cease the treatment should not be before 2nd birthday. Through three-month controls, the dose is increased by titration, with the aim of keeping T3 in the upper normal range. Due to the acceleration of metabolism (to normal), in order not to develop anemia and rickets, supplementation with iron, vitamin D, and calcium for 4–6 months is required.

6.2 Euthyroid sick syndrome

In more serious acute diseases (pneumonia, meningitis, tuberculosis, and sepsis), chronic diseases, consumptive conditions (tumors, starvation), and burns, the body conserves energy by reducing total T3 (by slowing deiodination from T4) and free T3 (translating it into reverse T3). Its decline is proportional to the severity of the disease. In severe long-term diseases, T4 also falls, whereas TSH usually remains normal because the feedback loop is maintained by T3 and reverse T3 together (hence they do not have a goiter). The condition is a physiological response and does not represent hypothyroidism (it is similar to the hibernation mechanism). It does not need to be treated with replacement therapy because it would worsen the underlying disease and passes with its cure, which is accompanied by a transient three-week increase in TSH up to a maximum of 20 mU/l.

6.3 Screening

Systematic search for congenital hypothyroidism by taking a blood sample from the heel and measuring TSH from each newborn is the basis for early initiation of therapy to prevent severe mental retardation. The first 2 days after birth (due to the lower ambient temperature compared to the intrauterine temperature and the moist skin of the newborn), TSH is high because it initiates the warming of the newborn. Therefore, it is important to draw blood only from the third day of life (in premature babies when they are 2 weeks old). Screening with T4 will detect newborns with secondary hypothyroidism also.

6.4 Neonatal hyperthyroidism

Neonatal hyperthyroidism is a rare and urgent condition that occurs as part of maternal hyperthyroidism and transplacental crossing of thyroid stimulating immunoglobulin (TSI). If the mother takes thyrostatic drugs (which also cross the placenta), the hyperthyroidism state in the newborn will appear only after a few days, when the drugs disappear from the circulation (but the stimulating antibodies are still present) and will last for about 2 months. The clinical picture is dominated by failure to thrive, diarrhea, tremor, exophthalmos, and tachycardia.

If neonatal hyperthyroidism is suspected, it is necessary to check the newborn (preferably around the fifth day) for free fractions of thyroid hormones (freeT3, freeT4), TSH and TSH-receptor antibodies in the blood (N: <15 U/l). It is important to note that normal values of total T3 and total T4 in the neonatal period are higher than those of adults, due to the higher concentration of TBG.

Neonatal hyperthyroidism is treated with thyrostatic drugs (thiamazole 0.5 mg/kg/day, divided into two doses) and propranolol (1–2 mg/kg/day, divided into two doses). Thyrotoxic storm requires the addition of iodine (Lugol solution 3×1 drop) and a shorter course of corticosteroids (methylprednisolone 2 mg/kg/day, divided into two doses).

Hyperfunction of multiple endocrine glands and self-activation of the intracellular G-unit is part of the clinical picture of McCune-Albright syndrome (they have unilateral hyperpigmented patches on the skin resembling coast of Maine).

7. Disorders of calcium metabolism

Calcium ions are an important for blood coagulation and neuromuscular activity, and it is a priority to provide it in the blood (not in bone tissue). Three hormones are involved in its regulation—parathyroid hormone, calcitonin, and D-hormone (calcitriol).

7.1 Transient neonatal hypocalcemia

Hypocalcemia includes values below 1.75 mmol/L (total calcium) or 0.9 mmol/L (ionic calcium) for a full-term newborn and 1.5 mmol/L (total calcium) or less than 0.75 mmol/L (ionic calcium) for a premature newborn.

Calcium easily crosses the placental barrier and is constantly available to the fetus, so its parathyroid glands are dormant. After birth, in the early neonatal period, transient hypocalcemia is possible, with a clinical picture of irritability, spasmophilia, and tetany, which can lead to spasm of the respiratory musculature, hypoxia, respiratory acidosis, and asphyxia. Correction of hypocalcemia is titrated only up to low normal level of serum calcium levels (about 2–2.2 mmol/l), so that borderline hypocalcemia is a continuous stimulus for the awakening of dormant parathyroid glands.

Hypocalcemia can be expected in children of pregnant women with diabetes (due to polyuria and increased excretion of calcium in the urine) and in children of pregnant women on anticonvulsant therapy (induction of hepatic enzymes that break down vitamin D).

Initially, for the correction of clinically manifested hypocalcemia, intravenous calcium preparations (20 mg/kg calculated as elemental calcium) are administered slowly over 30 min (prevention of bradycardia and local necrosis) every 6 h and are soon replaced by oral preparations (50 mg/kg/day, calculated as elemental calcium), with the introduction of vitamin D 400–1000 unit/day.

In hypocalcemic tetany, it is sometimes necessary to administer a continuous infusion of calcium at a dose of 1 mg/kg/h (calculated as elemental calcium) for 12–24 h.

Failure to respond adequately to treatment may indicate the need for correction of hypomagnesemia (10 mg/kg/day, calculated as elemental magnesium).

7.2 Hypercalcemia

Early age hypercalcemia (ionized calcium over 1.35 mmol/L) is usually associated with syndromes and specific conditions: Jansen metaphyseal chondrodysplasia, Williams syndrome (hypercalcemia, dwarf face, and aortic stenosis), subcutaneous fatty necrosis of the newborn, neonatal severe hyperparathyroidism (NSHPT) or IMAG syndrome (intrauterine growth retardation-IUGR + metaphyseal dysplasia + adrenal hypoplasia + genital anomalies). Hypercalcemia can also be the result of vitamin D intoxication or hyperparathyroidism.

Severe hypercalcemia from birth raises the suspicion of NSHPT, with hypophosphatemia, very high levels of parathyroid hormone, hypotonia, failure to thrive, respiratory distress, and bone demineralization, which causes deformities and fractures. The condition is caused by a mutation in the calcium-sensing receptor gene (CASR) localized on chromosome 3q21.1. Inheritance is more often autosomal recessive, less often autosomal dominant, and prevalence is unknown (rare). Differential diagnostic is familial hypocalciuric hypercalcemia (FHH), a condition that is most often asymptomatic, with milder hypercalcemia and lower levels of PTH. Treatment for NSHPT involves forced diuresis, bisphosphonates and calcimimetics (sinacalcet), with a low-calcium formula. Rarely does the solution may be a total parathyroidectomy.

When the total serum calcium is above 3 mmol/l, a clinical picture develops that includes lethargy, itching, nausea, vomiting, inappetence, weight loss, and polyuria.

Treatment of hypercalcemia includes hydration, diuretics of Henle's loop (furosemide), corticosteroids, calcitonin (1 IU/kg every 4–6 h), bisphosphonates (pamidronate infusion 1 mg/kg for 6 h), potassium preparation for the prevention of arrhythmia and cardiac arrest, phosphate administration, dialysis, and sinakalcet for NSHPT.

7.3 Benign hyperphosphatasia

A very common finding is a high alkaline phosphatase in relation to age (bone isoenzyme), with normal liver tests and calcium and phosphate in the blood. Spontaneously regresses by the sixth month of life.

8. Disorders of bone metabolism

8.1 Osteopenia of prematurity

Mineralization of bone tissue occurs mainly in the third trimester of fetal life, and osteopenia (reduction of the mineral component of bone tissue) occurs in premature newborns, between 10 and 16 weeks of age and is more common on breastfeeding. It carries a risk of spontaneous fractures in about 30% of newborns under 28 weeks of gestational age and in 55% of those born with a weight below 1000 g. The first predictors of this condition are a drop in phosphatemia (<1.5 mmol/L) around the third week of life and a flattened occipital bone. Vitamin D supplementation and oral calcium carbonate are useful in prevention and therapy.

8.2 Osteogenesis imperfecta

The disease belongs to the pathology of collagen, is manifested by repeated fractures to minor trauma ("glass bones"), and is inherited autosomal dominantly. Already at the neonatal age, indigo-blue sclera are present. A complication is a dissecting aneurysm. Hypercalciuria, high cross laps (collagen degradation product), and elevated alkaline phosphatase are present. Treatment involves orthopedic care and administration of bisphosphonates.

8.3 Hypermobility syndrome—general laxity

At least 20% of the population has hypermobility syndrome, which means weaker elastin and collagen fibers. It is inherited in an autosomal dominant manner. At an early age, the condition is manifested by cephalhematoma, intracranial hemorrhage, patent ductus, hydronephrosis, vesico-ureteral reflux, hypotonia, gastro-esophageal reflux, hernias, tendency to pneumothorax on artificial ventilation, craniotabes, slow closure of the fontanelles, intrapartum luxations and fractures, and immature hip architecture. Supplementation includes calcium, magnesium, vitamin D, ascorbic acid, and copper.

8.4 Rickets

The most common cause of rickets is vitamin D deficiency and usually manifests itself in the middle of infancy. In order to provide calcium in the blood for the coagulation cascade and neuromuscular tissues, parathyroid hormone ("spare vitamin D") increases and as a miner drills the bone and releases calcium and phosphate from hydroxyapatite. To prevent calcium phosphate from being deposited in soft tissues (it has a small solubility product), parathyroid hormone eliminates phosphate through the urine. In repair attempts, osteoblasts build bone and produce alkaline phosphatase. Thus, the laboratory picture of rickets includes low vitamin D, elevated parathyroid hormone, low phosphate in the serum, and elevated in the urine and high alkaline phosphatase, while calcium in the serum is normal, and when only the osteoid remains in the bones, then it also drops, causing tetany. The condition can be aggravated by celiac disease (due to malabsorption of liposoluble vitamins).

The clinical picture of rickets is manifested by soft bones and an attempt to repair them (craniotabes, large or long open fontanelles, X or O legs, costochondral rosaries, the wider wrist joint and later the caput quadratum, kyphoscoliosis, pectus carinatum or excavatum). An X-ray of the wrist shows a serrated calyx of radius.

Prophylaxis of rickets involves giving 400–1000 units of vitamin D per day (in continental climate also during the summer), especially when the infant is on breastfeeding (human milk does not have enough vitamin D since the human species entered closed spaces). Treatment involves giving 5000 units a day for about a month, with gradual introduction, to avoid "hungry bones."

8.5 Osteopetrosis

Albers-Schönberg is a severe "marble disease" due to osteoclast dysfunction, the absence of resorption of bone tissue and the transformation of bone into stones, including the medulla, leading to pancytopenia and consequent hepatosplenomegaly (extramedullary hematopoiesis). Growth is slowed down, and fractures are present already in the neonatal period (there is no collagen matrix-osteoid, and the bone is not resistant to traction and torsion). Gradually, neurological pathology develops due to craniosynostosis and nerve involvement. Alkaline phosphatase is elevated, and bone is excessively dense on osteodensitometry. There is no causal therapy, but one can try vitamin D (awakens dormant osteoclasts), corticosteroids (bone resorption), interferon (stimulates leukocytes), erythropoetin (for anemia), and bone marrow transplantation.

8.6 Other reasons for the abnormality of the skeletal system

Intrapartum fractures due to difficult childbirth, infantile myofibromatosis, fibrous dysplasia, congenital syphilis, hypophosphatasia (alkaline phosphatase deficiency), hypophosphatemic X-linked rickets, copper deficiency (it is necessary for the synthesis of elastin fibers), and chondrodystrophy (achondroplasia is easily recognized already at birth, due to rhizomelia and pronounced frontal prominences).

When a pathology of bone tissue is suspected, basic analyses include calcium, magnesium, phosphate, alkaline phosphatase, osteocalcin, P1NP, cross laps, vitamin D, parathyroid hormone and copper in serum, calciuria, X-ray, and osteodensitometry.

9. Glucose homeostasis disorders

9.1 Neonatal diabetes

Neonatal diabetes is a rare monogenic disease, with an incidence of 1:90,000 newborns. It occurs in the first 6 months of life as a permanent or transient form (disappears at 12 months of age, but reappears at 12 years of age or later). Clinical presentation includes IUGR, hypotonia, developmental delay, subsequent learning difficulties, epilepsy, and manifestations of diabetes (glycemia over 7 mmol/l after 4 h without food, with the possibility of ketoacidosis). It basically does not have an autoimmune mechanism, but rather a mutation of the KCNJ11, ABCC8 genes for ATP-sensitive potassium channel subunits or INS genes [6]. The ABCC8 gene provides instructions for the synthesis of the SUR1 protein, a subunit of the pancreatic ATP-sensitive potassium channel (sulfonylurea receptor). The closing of this channel opens a flood-gate for insulin release. A mutation in the ABCC8 gene can cause congenital hyperinsulinism or neonatal diabetes. Mutations in other responsible genes have also been described. After genetic testing, the type of therapy (insulin or oral sulfonylureas) is recommended.

Sometimes neonatal diabetes occurs within the syndrome (Wolcot-Rallison, immune dysregulation-polyendocrinopathy-enteropathy-X-linked IPEX, Roger). The onset of the disease is usually sudden with hyperglycemia and pronounced dehydration, low levels of C-peptides, low insulinemia with massive glycosuria, up to ketoacidosis.

9.2 Transient hyperglycemia of prematurity

Although preterm birth is known to be associated with hypoglycemia, SGA and extremely low weight infants (ELBW) are prone to hyperglycemia (over 7 mmol/L in plasma and over 8.3 mmol/L in whole blood), possibly by a central mechanism (hypothalamus), due to deficient proinsulin synthesis, immaturity of the glucose transporters (GLUT) system, or due to an excessive response of antiinsular hormones. It occurs within the first 10 days and lasts 2–3 days. Hyperglycemia increases the risk of cerebral hemorrhage (due to osmotic polyuria and consecutive hypernatremia), necrotizing enterocolitis (NEC), retinopathy of prematurity (ROP), and bronchopulmonary dysplasia.

Incorrect administration of intravenous fluids or parenteral nutrition with higher glucose infusion rates is a frequent iatrogenic contributing factor for hyperglycemia.

Treatment involves reduction of caloric intake to 50 kcal/kg/day in the first days and administering insulin in low doses when necessary (0.01 units/kg/h).

Hyperglycemia is seen also after treatment with dexamethasone, dopamine, or caffeine.

9.3 Neonatal hypoglycemia

The largest consumer of glucose (energy) in the body is brain tissue, especially at an early age, when it requires energy for both function and the growth and differentiation of brain tissue. In the case of hypoglycemia, a pathological EEG appears when the glycemia drops to 2.6 mmol/L, so this value is generally accepted as low for full-term newborns, infants, children, and adults. Lower values can cause brain damage. It seems that the immature neurons of premature infants and the altered neurons of the epileptogenic focus of larger children are capable of using ketones, so they tolerate glycemia half of the cited value −1.3 mmol/l.

The clinical picture of hypoglycemia of neonatal age is nonspecific and is manifested by apnea, cyanosis, irritability, tremor, twitches, high-pitched cry, lethargy, and hypotonia.

Hypoglycemia in the early neonatal period is most often caused by high energy expenditure or poor food intake. In premature infants, the iatrogenic cause of hypoglycemia is common—insufficient intake of energy products by infusion (1 g of glucose is only 4 kcal). Rarely, reasons for hypoglycemia are metabolic diseases (von Gierke, maple syrup urine disease (MSUD), galactosemia) and endocrine pathology (hypopituitarism, hemorrhage in both adrenal glands). Taking propranolol during pregnancy in a newborn causes transient hypoglycemia.

Hyperinsulinemia is characterized by the absence of the formation of ketone bodies in hypoglycemia, since insulin protects adipose tissue from lipolysis. Underlying conditions with hyperinsulinism include Beckwith-Wiedemann, Sotos syndrome, a child of a pregnant woman with diabetes, and others.

Prevention and treatment of neonatal hypoglycemia includes early breastfeeding, initial administration of 5–10% glucose or dextrose gel orally, increase in the number of meals, avoidance of intravenous bolus of hypertonic glucose, and administration of a continuous infusion of 5–10–12.5% glucose (6 mg/kg/min). Refractory conditions (hypoglycemia that is not resolved within the first 72 h and does not improve even with the administration of 12 mg/kg/min of glucose) demands hydrocortisone IV 10 mg/kg/day (divided into 2–4 doses), glucagon i.v./i.m. 0.3 mg/kg/pro dosi, adrenalin s.c. 0.01 mg/kg/pro dosi, diazoxide IV 10 ml/kg/day (divided into three doses), and partial or subtotal pancreatectomy is the last resort, after which diabetes can occur.

10. Disorders of adrenal gland

The adrenal axis is the most important because, through ACTH and cortisol, it provides energy through gluconeogenesis and enables a proper stress response. Therefore, evolutionarily, ACTH basophilic pituicytes are the most resistant to infections, toxins, and radiation.

10.1 Congenital adrenal hyperplasia (CAH)

The most common cause of CAH is a partial or total deficiency of the enzyme 21-hydroxylase, necessary for the synthesis of both cortisol and aldosterone. The disease is inherited in an autosomal recessive manner. Low cortisol by feedback mechanism leads to the tide of ACTH in utero and stimulates the fasciculata zone, but also to some extent the reticularis zone, leading to their hyperplasia. Flood of precursors (17-OH-progesterone) improves the production of cortisol but diverts them to androgen pathway, thus finally forming the clinical picture (concomitant hypocorticism due to insufficient cortisol production and hypercorticism due to increased androgen production). Undetected and untreated, it can trigger central puberty.

Girls are born with clitoridomegalia (clitoral length > 1 cm and width > 0.6 cm) [7] and/or labial fusion (sometimes resembling a boy with cryptorchidism), and boys with hyperpigmentation of the scrotum. The capacitance of the stress response in these newborns is insufficient (cortisol in stress should rise 2–10 times).

The same enzyme (21-hydroxylase) is necessary in small amounts for the synthesis of aldosterone and in large amounts for the synthesis of cortisol. Therefore, the partial defect of the enzyme is manifested only by the insufficient production of cortisol (possible hypoglycemia), and only the absolute one affects the aldosterone pathway. Then, due to the deficiency of aldosterone in the newborn period, there is also a loss of salt (sodium) through the kidneys, sweat glands and intestines (vomiting and diarrhea), and the retention of potassium (sodium is low, and potassium is high in the blood). Metabolic acidosis (due to hyperkalemia) and hypoglycemia (due to low cortisolemia) may occur. The condition is urgent because dehydration and hyperkalemia can cause a fatal course. A "boy with cryptorchidism," dehydration (vomiting and diarrhea), hyponatremia, and hyperkalemia may be a female newborn with CAH, due to a total deficiency of 21-hydroxylase. CAH could also include inspissated bile syndrome.

The condition cannot be detected by ultrasound. Laboratory tests show low borderline cortisol (cortisol levels should be at least 220 nmol/L; there is usually no circadian rhythm in the first month), elevated cortisol precursor 17-hydroxyprogesterone (17-OH-P), and high ACTH. With the application of tetracosactide-cosyntropin (the active part of the ACTH molecule)—Synacthen test, the level of cortisol does not double, and the level of 17-OH-P rises even more. In 24 h of urine, there are high levels of 17-KS (17-ketosteroids—the final metabolite of androgens), elevated pregnantriol (the final metabolite of 17-OH-P), and dehydroepiandrosterone (DHEA—a weak androgen, specific for the adrenal gland). Involvement of aldosterone pathway will bring hyponatremia (hypovolemia) and hyperkalemia.

Therapy is lifelong and comprises hydrocortisone at initial dose 15 $mg/m^2/24$ h, divided into three asymmetric doses (the evening dose is the highest to suppress the night tide of ACTH). In phases of stress (infections, endoscopy, and surgery), the dose should be increased 2–5 times, in order to mimic the normal stress response. In case of absolute enzyme deficiency (salt loss syndrome), it is necessary to introduce a mineralocorticosteroid (fludrocortisone) at a dose of 0.05–0.1 mg/day (up to a maximum of 0.3 mg/day). Controls are carried out every 3 months, through laboratory monitoring (ACTH, cortisol, 17-OH-P, and DHEA-S 1 h after morning dosage) and clinical monitoring (growth, signs of virilization, and weight).

In crises with salt loss, in addition to fludrocortisone, infusions of glucose and saline, the intake of 1–2 g of salt per day, and the intravenous administration of hydrocortisone are necessary.

In the long term, treatment includes clitoroplasty in infancy, lifelong corticosteroid replacement therapy—hydrocortisone, increasing the dose of glucocorticoid 2–5 times during intercurrent disease or surgical intervention (imitation of the stress response), fludrocortisone (0.05–0.1 mg/day) as needed (in absolute enzyme deficiency and salt loss syndrome), monitoring of growth, bone age, androgens, and 17-hydroxyprogesterone and DHEA-S in the blood. Underdosed glucocorticoid replacement therapy leads to high ACTH and androgenic excess, which accelerates bone maturation and gives a lower definitive height, while an overdose slows down growth.

Incidence of CAH is 1 in 10,000 newborns, and in some countries screening for CAH has been introduced. Prenatal diagnosis is sought when the family already has a child with congenital adrenal hyperplasia, and if the fetus is female, dexamethasone may be given to a pregnant woman to reduce fetal ACTH and the degree of virilization of the fetus.

The second most common variant of congenital adrenal hyperplasia (1:100,000) is 11-betahydroxylase deficiency, when there is an accumulation of deoxycorticosterone (DOC) with consecutive salt retention, hypertension in two-thirds of cases, and virilization.

Rare condition 3-beta-hydroxysteroid dehydrogenase deficiency means decreased hormone production in all three zones (and a spike in ACTH). There is no translation of pregnenolone to progesterone in the glomerulose zone, no translation of 17-alpha-hydroxy-pregnenolone to 17-alpha-hydroxyprogesterone in the fasciculata zone, and no translation of DHEA into androstenedione in the reticular zone. The condition is manifested by hyponatremia-hyperkalemia, insufficient masculinization (hypospadias, gynecomastia) in boys, and moderate clitoral hypertrophy and/or labial fusion in girls (due to DHEA tide). A mild form of this condition is seen at a later age and is recognized by acne, hirsutism, polycystic ovaries, and acceleration of linear growth/osseous maturity.

10.2 Hypocorticism (adrenal insufficiency)

The most common reasons for hypocorticism at an early age are X-linked adrenal hypoplasia, adrenoleukodystrophy, IMAG syndrome, Wolman syndrome (thesaurism due to acid lipase deficiency in lysosomes), and hemorrhage in both adrenal glands.

10.3 Hemorrhage in the adrenal gland

The fetal adrenal glands are relatively large and, with the normal presentation of the fetus, are projected onto the rib arches of the mother. When obstetrician is pressing on them during expulsion of the fetus, intraadrenal hemorrhage (often bilateral) can occur, which is detected by ultrasonography. After 10–14 days, it often takes the form of a chocolate cyst, and later the hematoma is resorbed, organized, and, usually, calcified (visible as a starry shadow under the diaphragm, on an X-ray).

Suspicion of adrenal hemorrhage may be aroused by anamnesis (difficult childbirth), examination (icteric coloration because of hyperbilirubinemia due to hematoma resorption), and hypoglycemia (cortisol deficiency). Cortisolemia is low (below 220 nmol/l) and accompanied by a spike in ACTH, which requires the introduction of hydrocortisone replacement therapy in an asymmetric arrangement (the morning dose should be the highest, mimicking the circadian profile of cortisol), but not at the full dose, so that borderline high ACTH contributes to tissue restoration after hematoma resorption. Corticosteroids are usually given for at least 2 weeks in continuo, then every second (later third) day, with cortisol levels checked on empty days, and then given only in stressful situations (intercurrent infection, surgical interventions). Minimal morning cortisolemia for stressful days should be at least 220 nmol/l. Due to the constant lighting in the hospitals and the immaturity of circadian rhythms in neonatal period and early infancy, afternoon cortisolemia at 4 pm is unnecessary. If needed, to stimulate the fascicular zone and revitalize the glands, tetracosactide-cosyntropine Synacthen can be applied (do not administer Synacthen depot at an early age, due to possible hemolysis because of benzyl alcohol). Lower sodium (along with higher potassium) and very low arterial pressure speak for a lesion of the glomerulosis zone. The prognosis is generally good, and the capacitance of the fascicular zone can be checked by the Synacthen test.

Without treatment and supervision, the combination of hypocortisolemia and intercurrent infection or surgery can be fatal in these children.

10.4 Hypercorticism

Cushing's syndrome is rare in children and has pituitary (80%) or adrenal (20%) origin, with various pathology in the background [8]. The clinical picture includes centripetal obesity, hypertension, hirsutism, stretch marks, plethora, and cessation of growth. The laboratory profile includes polyglobulia, leukocytosis, lymphocytopenia, decreased eosinophil count, hyperglycemia, hypogammaglobulinemia, hypernatremia, hypokalemia, borderline hypocalcemia, increase in creatinine, increased blood coagulability, absence of an afternoon drop in cortisolemia (applicable in later infancy, when endocrine axes are established), and a pathological short dexamethasone test. Therapy is surgical.

11. Disorders of sex differentiation

The genital system has complicated development. In each embryo, there are structures of both sexes—Müller's ducts (female structures) and Wolff's channels (male structures). Which structure will develop depends primarily on genetic factors.

Sex is usually determined by sex chromosomes. Each individual must have at least one X-chromosome to survive, as is the case with Turner syndrome (45,X). A normal female has two X chromosomes. An excess of X chromosomes ("super women") leads to poorer mental performance, logorrhea, and fertility disorders, and in men (47,XXY) it induces feminine somatic characteristics. An excess Y-chromosome (47,XYY) produces a higher growth rate and learning difficulties.

The chromosomal and phenotypic sexes are not always congruent. Thus, XX people can have a male (XX male) and XY female phenotype (Swyer syndrome), depending on the location or mutation of SRY (a group of genes on the sex region of the Y-chromosome), responsible for the synthesis of TDF (testicle-determining factor), which translates the indifferent gonad into the testicle.

To become a biologically real man, three key points in successive order are required: intact SRY, 5-alpha reductase (converts testosterone to dihydrotestosterone) and normal architecture of androgen receptors (**Figure 3**). If only one is missing, the phenotype will be female.

11.1 Pathology of SRY

If SRY is mutated, testis determining factor (TDF) will be missing, and the streak gonad and female phenotype will develop, with karyotype 46,XY (Swyer syndrome). Early extirpation of rudimentary gonads, due to possible neoplasms, and subsequent administration of estrogen to induce secondary sexual signs (puberty) prevent depression and osteoporosis. Mosaicism 45,X/46,XY is called mixed gonadal dysgenesis.

SRY is normally located on the Y chromosome, but by translocation during meiosis ("grasshopper"), it can be found on the X chromosome of the father's sperm, and by fusing with the egg, XX-male (de la Chapelle syndrome) will result. These male newborns have a micropenis, and later infertility and decreased libido. The condition could be detected prenatally by comparing the result of early amniocentesis (karyotype 46, XX) with fetal ultrasonography depicting penis.

11.2 Pathology of the enzyme 5-α reductase

Testosterone is responsible for the development of a male internal genitalia. Enzyme 5α-reductase converts it to more powerful androgen DHT (dihydrotestosterone) which is responsible for the formation of the external male genitalia.

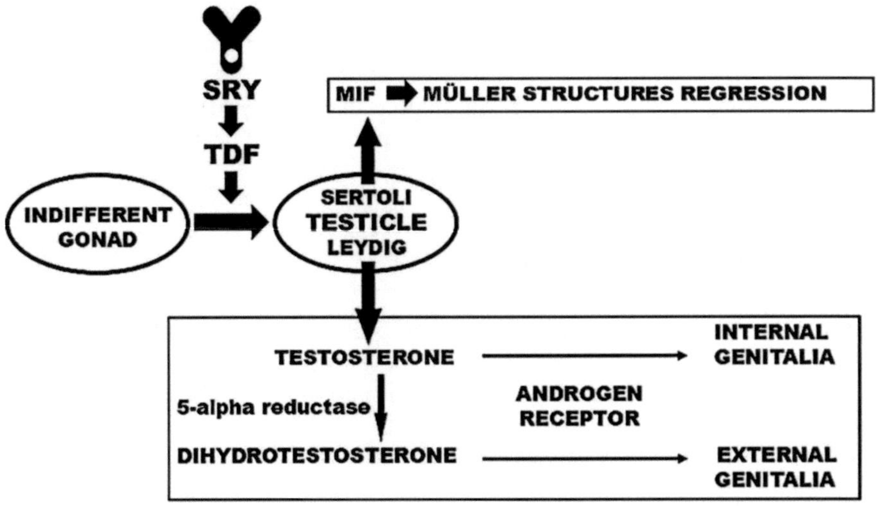

Figure 3.
Three key points for male development-SRY, 5-alpha reductase, and androgen receptors.

If the enzyme 5α-reductase is absent or ineffective, there is not enough DHT in the male fetus, only the internal genital develops, and the newborn is declared female (testicles are retained, with high testosterone to DHT plasma ratio).[3] When, at puberty (usually at the age of 12), high concentration of testosterone acts like DHT, the growth of the penis and the descensus of the testicles occurs. The condition is popularly referred to as penis at 12 (Spanish guevedoce) and includes microgenitosomia, scrotum bifidum, and bisexual orientation (higher incidence in the Dominican Republic, Papua New Guinea, Turkey).

11.3 Pathology of androgen receptors

Defective androgen receptors disable the action of testosterone and DHT, regardless of the normal male karyotype (46,XY), the presence of testicles, testosterone production, and the presence of 5-alpha reductase (which converts testosterone to dihydrotestosterone leading to their normal ratio).

The condition is called androgen insensitivity syndrome (AIS) and is present in three forms, depending on the degree of alteration in the architecture of androgen receptors:

Mild androgen insensitivity syndrome (MAIS) cannot be recognized at birth. Later, a high level of testosterone is detected (it is not spent on the receptors), but the hairiness is less pronounced (weaker beard).

Partial androgen insensitivity syndrome (PAIS)—Reifenstein syndrome is manifested by ambivalent genitalia at birth, and ultrasonography reveals intra-abdominal testicles[4].

Complete androgen insensitivity syndrome (CAIS) leads to bilateral inguinal hernias at birth, in which there are actually testicles—the image of a female newborn

[3] Differential diagnosis is AIS (CAIS and PAIS).

[4] Differential diagnosis is 5-alfa reductase deficiency.

with hernias should always raise the suspicion of androgen insensitivity syndrome. The testicles produce testosterone (which is not utilized at the receptors) and is converted by adipose tissue into estradiol and at puberty a typical female phenotype develops with formed breasts, but without axillary and pubic hair. These individuals are somewhat higher and usually refer because of primary amenorrhea. The old name of the condition is testicular feminization. The testicles can malignantly alter and must be surgically removed. Later, estrogen replacement therapy is introduced to induce sexual development (there is no need for a progesterone component, since they do not have a uterus). Rokitansky syndrome is an anomaly that occurs in female individuals of karyotype 46,XX (underdevelopment or absence of the vagina and/or uterus) and does not belong to this entity.

11.4 Micropenis

The micropenis is defined by the dimension outside the erection less than 2.5 cm (width less than 0.9 cm) at neonatal age (average is 3.5 cm), less than 2 cm in a premature newborn GS at 34 weeks or less than 1.5 cm in a premature newborn GS at 30 weeks. This may indicate a deficiency of gonadotropins. Associated hypoglycemia (below 2.6 mmol/l) due to ACTH (cortisol) deficiency favors panhypopituitarism. If the micropenis is neither a sign of panhypopituitarism, nor hypertrophic clitoris of a female child with virilization (congenital adrenal hyperplasia), only after obtaining the male karyotype (46,XY), androgen, or gonadotropin treatment should be applied. Intermittent i.m. testosterone enanthate for penis enlargement can be administered: 25–50 mg three times, with an interval of 4–6 weeks [9]. Topical transdermal DHT gel can be used as well.

11.5 Cryptorchidism

When testicles are hidden and cannot be found by palpation, ultrasonography, MRI, or Primogonyl test (a rise in testosterone level after administration of gonadotropins) should be performed. The undescended testicles can be graded as intra-abdominal, inguinal, or retractile. Only the migratory (mobile) testicle does not require therapy.

Bilateral testicular retention is part of the clinical picture of certain syndromes (Prader-Willi-Labhart, Silver-Russell, Noonan, Beckwith-Wiedemann, etc.).

In full-term (male) newborns, testicular retention (mostly unilateral) is present in 3.4%. At the age of 1 year, 0.7% of boys still do not have complete descension of both testicles. After the age of two, testicular retention carries a risk of damage to the germinal epithelium, and at the age of 8, the risk of tumors in middle age increases significantly. Therefore, cryptorchidism needs to be resolved by the first, and no later than the second birthday (the examination begins after the sixth month of life, since later the chance of spontaneous descension is minimal).

Hormone treatment is less successful [10] and involves intramuscular administration of gonadotropin (hCG) or nasal administration of gonadorelin (LH-RH) or both drugs successively or buserelin (Gn-RH agonist). In infancy, 250 IU of hCG twice weekly i.m. for 5 weeks (10 injections in total) or gonadorelin 1.2 mg (3 × 0.4 mg) daily nasally for 28 days or buserelin 20 mcg daily nasally for 28 days is given. All of these regimens lead to a local tide of testosterone from Leydig cells, which elongates the funiculus spermaticus (without the systemic effect that would result from testosterone injections).

Side effects of hormone treatment of an undescended testicle are mild and transient, and the only contraindications are previous surgery of the groin (scars), ectopic testicle, or associated hernia.

In case of failure of hormone therapy or even before its application (depending on the position of the testicles), the child is referred to a urologist for orchidopexy. During the intervention, ectopic adrenal cortex can sometimes be found. It is always yellow in color and does not contain elements of the medulla, which has another embryonic origin. Synthetic analogue of gonadotropin-releasing hormone (GnRH) buserelin is recommended for 6 months after orchidopexy (10 mcg every other day nasally).

11.6 Testes vanishing syndrome (congenital anorchia, testicular regression syndrome)

Disappeared testicles (incidence 1/1250 males) refer to a normal penis without testicles [11, 12], which in the late fetal period were destroyed by a probable autoimmune process (then the first differential diagnosis is congenital adrenal hyperplasia in a female child).

11.7 Hermaphroditism

It refers to the presence of both types of gonads, through the form of the ovotestis or ovary on one side and the testicle on the other. It can be confirmed in the laboratory by measuring the levels of testosterone and estradiol before and after the administration of gonadotropins—there is a raise in both hormones.

The team for diagnosing and monitoring newborns with sex differentiation problems (**Table 2**) consists of an endocrinologist, a urologist, gynecologist, geneticist, and a psychologist later in life. Initial examination in ambivalent genitalia includes karyotype, hormonal status (17-OH-progesterone, Primogonyl test), and ultrasonography of the internal genitalia.[5]

11.8 Premature thelarche

Isolated breast enlargement, with no other signs of sexual development) is seen in the neonatal and infant periods. The first differential diagnosis is precocious puberty, which could be excluded by normal length and bone age. It spontaneously regresses by the end of the second year of life [13].

11.9 Congenital ovarian cysts

Often detected by chance in the neonatal period, it can be diagnosed intrauterine by ultrasonography. Incidence is 1/2500 female newborns [14–16]. Their formation is influenced by high levels of hCG from placenta, and they usually spontaneously regress in the first 3–6 months of life, especially if they are below 4 cm in diameter [17]. They are rarely malignant, but it is necessary to monitor estradiol, hCG, and alpha-fetoprotein as tumor markers. Possible complications are intestinal obstruction, hemorrhage, torsion (in cysts over 4 cm), and rupture, when surgical intervention is necessary.

---

[5] Testicle is like chestnut (smooth surface), while ovarium looks like walnut (bumpy).

DOI: http://dx.doi.org/10.5772/intechopen.1010285

Kariotype	**Pathology**	**Phenotype (external genitalia)**	**Diagnosis**
46,XY	SRY	Female	Swyer syndrome
46,XY	5-alpha reductase	Female → Male	Penis at 12
46,XY	Androgen receptor	Male	MAIS
		Ambiguous	PAIS
		Female	CAIS
46,XX	Sperm meiosis	Male	XX male
46,XX	21-hydroxylase	Virilization	CAH

Table 2.
Sex differentiation pathology.

12. Water metabolism

12.1 Diabetes insipidus

Diabetes insipidus occurs due to insufficient secretion of antidiuretic hormone (ADH) from the neurohypophysis (central type) or refractory renal tubules (nephrogenic form). In both cases, polyuria and consecutive polydipsia occur. Central diabetes insipidus occurs after head trauma, intracranial tumors or surgery, and histiocytosis of bone or brain tissue.

The basic diagnostics include a thirst test, which lasts about 8–12 h in the infant period. To definitively distinguish between central and nephrogenic insipid diabetes, the test is completed with the administration of ADH (DDAVP), when the condition will improve only with the central form of the disease. Potomania at an early age is usually the result of the infant being put to sleep by giving fluids during the night.

12.2 Syndrome of inadequate secretion of ADH (SIADH)

It is normal for ADH to be secreted in states of dehydration. However, in some conditions (in practice, most often with birth asphyxia, meningitis, pneumonia, or subarachnoid and subdural hemorrhage), the level of this hormone increases [18], resulting in fluid retention, dilutionary hyponatremia (below 135 mmol/L), decreased or normal urea, serum hypoosmolality (below 275 mOsmol/kg), and urine hyperosmolarity (over 1000 mOsmol/kg). Therapy is fluid restriction.

Differential diagnosis includes hypotonic dehydration (hyponatremia is present, but urea is normal or higher due to prerenal azotemia), cerebral salt wasting syndrome (CSWS), which occurs shortly after trauma (subarachnoid hematoma) or head surgery (due to tumor or hydrocephalus), when hyponatremia and hypernatriuria, an increase in urea and polyuria, are present.

13. Endocrine disruptors

Chemical agents that interfere with hormone synthesis or the endocrine process are called disruptors. Most often they belong to pollutants (petrochemicals, pesticides) or analgesics, and less often they are natural substances. They can lead to disorders in sex differentiation, hypothyroidism, cryptorchism, tumorigenesis, or early puberty [19, 20].

14. Conclusion

The transition from fetal life to independent existence is a stressful event for the newborn, requiring significant adaptation and intricate hormone balance. At the neonatal age, the most important are the adrenal and thyroid axis. The first one provides energy through cortisol, builds up blood volume through aldosterone, while androgens trigger puberty at a later age, when the activity of the gonadal axis is most pronounced (3s—sugar, salt, sex). The thyroid axis makes humans homeotherms and determines the rate of metabolic processes. In the spectrum of sex-differentiation pathology, if any of the key-points for male development is missing (SRY, 5-alpha reductase, proper androgen receptors), female phenotype will ensue. Newborns have polyphasic sleep pattern, and their three-hour ultradian rhythm (related to breast-feeding) becomes circadian around 6 months of age. Knowledge of the semiotics of endocrine disorders and the correct interpretation of laboratory results at an early age contributes to the right and prompt decision, life-saving treatment and could have a lifelong consequence.

Appendix

See **Tables 3** and **4**.

Syndrome	Condition
Beckwith-Wiedemann	Omphalocele, visceromegaly, hypoglycemia, and large newborn
McCune-Albright	Hyperpigmentation, endocrine hyperfunction
Noonan	Pterygium colli (webbed neck), pulmonary stenosis, and undescended testicles
Prader-Willi-Labhart	Hypotonia, failure to thrive
Silver-Russell	Large triangular head (impression of hydrocephalus), SGA, and clinodactyly V
Sotos	Gigantism
Turner	Puffy feet, pterygium colli (webbed neck), low set ears, and low back hairline
Williams	Hypercalcemia, dwarf face, aortic stenosis
De Morsier (SOD)	Nystagmus, strabismus

Table 3.
Syndromes with endocrine pathology recognizable in the neonatal period.

Signs	Condition to consider
Midline anomalies (micropenis, septo-optic dysplasia, cheilognathopalatschisis, and central incisor)	Panhypopituitarism
Micropenis	XX male (de la Chapelle syndrome)
Micropenis with cryptorchism	Enlarged clitoris in female newborn with CAH
Pterygium colli (webbed neck)	Turner syndrome
Bilateral hernia in female newborn	AIS
Oedema + prolonged jaundice + hypothermia + bradycardia + enlarged posterior fontanel	Hypothyroidism
Clitoral hypertrophy, hyperkaliemia, inspissated bile syndrome	CAH
Hyperbilirubinemia	Hypothyroidism, adrenal hemorrhage
Hypercalcemia	Williams syndrome, NSHPT, hypervitaminosis D, and Jansen syndrome
Hypoglycemia	Newborn of diabetic mother, panhypopituitarism, and Beckwith-Wiedemann syndrome
Hyponatremia	SIADH, hypotonic dehydration, CAH, CSWS, hypoaldosteronism, and pseudohypoaldosteronism

Table 4.
Clinical signs in neonatal endocrinology.

Author details

Dragan Katanić
Faculty of Medicine, Novi Sad, Serbia

*Address all correspondence to: dr.dragan.katanic@gmail.com

References

[1] Gluckman PD, Bassett N, Ball KT. The functional maturation of the somatotropic axis in the perinatal period. In: Künzel W, Jensen A, editors. The Endocrine Control of the Fetus. Berlin: Springer-Verlag; 1988. pp. 201-209. ISBN 0-387-18334-5

[2] Cabral S, LeBouc Y. Retard de croissance a debut intra-uterin. In: Limal JM, editor. Endocrinologie Périnatale. Rueil-Malmaison: Doin-Groupe Liaisons; 2005. pp. 46-56. ISBN-13: 978-2704011896. Available from: https://lib.fmpm.uca.ma/lib/opac_css/index.php?lvl=publisher_see&id=388; https://promotion-sante-guadeloupe.centredoc.org/index.php?lvl=publisher_see&id=165

[3] Fenton TR, Kim JH. A systematic review and meta-analysis to revise the Fenton growth chart for preterm infants. BMC Pediatrics. 2013;**13**(1):59. DOI: 10.1186/1471-2431-13-59

[4] Morris RK, Johnstone E, Lees C. Investigation and care of a small-for-gestational-age fetus and a growth restricted fetus (green-top guideline No. 31). BJOG: An International Journal of Obstetrics & Gynaecology. 2024;**131**:e31-e80. DOI: 10.1111/1471-0528.17814

[5] Lyle AN, Pokuah F, Dietzen DJ, et al. Current state of pediatric reference intervals and the importance of correctly describing the biochemistry of child development: A review. JAMA Pediatrics. 2022;**176**(7):699-714. DOI: 10.1001/jamapediatrics.2022.0794

[6] Katanic D, Vorgučin I, Hattersley A, et al. A successful transition to sulfonylurea treatment in male infant with neonatal diabetes caused by the novel abcc8 gene mutation and three years follow-up. Diabetes Research and Clinical Practice. 2017;**129**:59-61. DOI: 10.1016/j.diabres.2017.04.021

[7] Oberfield SE, Mondok A, Shahrivar F, et al. Clitoral size in full-term infants. American Journal of Perinatology. 1989;**6**(4):453-454. DOI: 10.1055/s-2007-999638

[8] Katanić D, Kafka D, Živojinov M, et al. Primary pigmented nodular adrenocortical disease: Literature review and case report of a 6-year-old boy. Journal of Pediatric Endocrinology and Metabolism. 2017;**30**(5):603-609. DOI: 10.1515/jpem-2016-0249

[9] Cezarino BN, Lopes RI, Machado MG, et al. Micropenis. Revista de Medicina (São Paulo). 2018;**97**(3):308-313. DOI: 10.11606/issn.1679-9836.v97i3p308-313

[10] Sumfest JM. Cryptorchidism Treatment & Management. 2014. Available from: https://emedicine.medscape.com/article/438378-treatment [Accessed: 2 October 2025]

[11] Jayawickreme KP, Hashim R, Antonypillai CN. A rare case of bilateral vanishing testicle syndrome. Sri Lanka Journal of Diabetes Endocrinology and Metabolism. 2023;**14**(2):51-57. DOI: 10.4038/sjdem.v14i2.7495

[12] Hombalkar DP, Gurav N, Khan P, et al. Vanishing testis syndrome: Report of two cases. Journal of Clinical and Diagnostic Research: JCDR. 2014;**8**(8):ND03-ND04. DOI: 10.7860/JCDR/2014/8315.4715

[13] Khokhar A, Mojica A. Premature thelarche. Pediatric Annals. 2018;**47**(1):e12-e15. DOI: 10.3928/19382359-20171214-01

[14] Llorens Salvador R, Sangüesa Nebot C, Pacheco Usmayo A, et al. Neonatal ovarian cysts: Ultrasound assessment and differential diagnosis. Radiología. 2017;**59**(1):31-39. DOI: 10.1016/j.rxeng.2016.10.001

[15] Rohayem J, Alexander EC, Heger S, et al. Mini-puberty, physiological and disordered: Consequences, and potential for therapeutic replacement. Endocrine Reviews. 2024;**45**(4):460-492. DOI: 10.1210/endrev/bnae003

[16] Bayramoğlu E, Erdeve ŞS, Derinkuyu BE, et al. Clitoromegaly caused by ovarian stimulation in a preterm newborn: Ovarian hyperstimulation syndrome of preterm babies. The Turkish Journal of Pediatrics. 2020;**62**(6):1088-1093. DOI: 10.24953/turkjped.2020.06.022

[17] Vorgučin I, Katanić D, Kovačević B, et al. Preterm ovarian hyperstimulation syndrome: A clinical presentation of three cases. Journal of Neonatal Biology. 2018;**4**(1):7-14. DOI: 10.15436/2380-5595.18.1802

[18] Gagandeep V, Vidhya PS. Syndrome of inappropriate antidiuretic hormone secretion in neonates with birth asphyxia at tertiary care centre. International Journal of Contemporary Pediatrics. 2019;**6**(6):2549-2553. DOI: 10.18203/2349-3291.ijcp20194732

[19] Citron K, Murthy DB, Shah B. Endocrine-disrupting chemicals in children. Pediatrics in Review. 2024;**45**(2):111-115. DOI: 10.1542/pir.2022-005725

[20] Gore AC. Endocrine-Disrupting Chemicals. Totowa: Humana Press; 2007. ISBN 978-1-61737-795-2

Chapter 6

Etiological Evaluation and Management of Neonatal Seizures

Duygu Acar

Abstract

Neonatal seizures can be a clinical sign of a central nervous system disorder. Incidences of seizures range from 1.5 to 5.5 per 1000 in newborns. Seizures can be seen all periods of neonates, but most often occur within the first week of life. The most common cause of seizure is neonatal encephalopathy and hypoxic ischemic encephalopathy. There are two types of seizures: electro-clinical and electrographic-only. Clinical types of neonatal seizures are focal clonic, focal tonic, myoclonic, epileptic spasms, and sequential seizures. Subclinical or silent seizures are now termed electrographic-only seizures. It can be hard to distinguish non-seizure paroxysmal events from seizures in the neonatal period. Multi-channel video continuous EEG (cEEG) monitoring is the gold standard for neonatal seizure diagnosis. In the management of neonatal seizures, the initial steps involve controlling the newborn's airway, breathing, and circulation. Phenobarbital is still the first choice of initial antiseizure medication therapy drug for infants.

Keywords: neonatal seizures, electroencephalography, anti-seizure medication, phenobarbital, neonatal epilepsy, hypoxic-ischemic encephalopathy

1. Introduction

Neonatal seizures are one of the most common emergency neurological events in the early period after birth.

Neonatal seizure is an important clinical condition in this period. Seizures are usually have a potentially treatable etiology and should be evaluated immediately to determine the cause and to start therapy for the specific etiology. As soon as possible, seizures must be solved because they may adversely affect the newborn's vital signs or contribute to further brain injury.

The incidence of seizures ranges from 1.5 to 5.5 per 1000 in newborns [1–3]. Seizure frequency increases as gestational age and birth weight decreases [4–6]. Also, the frequency of seizures is higher in the neonatal period, compared to whole of life.

Approximately 85% of neonatal seizures have a specific identifiable etiology and called acute provoked seizures [7–11]. Formerly, acute provoked seizures are named as acute symptomatic seizures. Epilepsy syndromes are relatively rare in this period (15%) [12]. Previously called benign familial neonatal epilepsy, today called self-limited neonatal epilepsy syndrome, it may have a genetic etiology and mostly negative work-up, well appearing neonates. Newborn with abnormal brain imaging or abnormal neurologic examination has probably early infantile developmental and epileptic encephalopathy that has poor prognosis. Early infantile developmental and epileptic encephalopathy is previously called early myoclonic encephalopathy and Ohtahara syndrome. Etiological causes of acute provoked seizures can be listed as follows:

- Neonatal encephalopathy due to perinatal asphyxia
- Structural brain injuries, like ischemic and hemorrhagic stroke
- Metabolic abnormalities (most often hypoglycemia)
- Infections of the central nervous system such as meningitis and encephalitis

2. Clinical features

There are two types of seizures in newborns: electroclinical seizures and electrographic-only seizures. Electrographic-only seizures were previously named subclinical "or "silent" seizures and has no clinical signs with characterized presence of an electrographic seizure on electroencephalography (EEG) [10, 11, 13, 14].

Because of newborn's immature brain, neonatal seizures are not generalized [11]. Clinical events are mostly focal clonic, focal tonic, and some types of myoclonic and epileptic spasms.

Focal clonic seizures: slow repetitive and rhythmic contractions of specific muscle groups of the limbs, face, or trunk are characteristic of focal clonic seizures. Each contraction consists of a close alignment with the EEG seizure pattern. Focal clonic seizures can be unifocal or multifocal. Multifocal clonic seizures may exhibit clonic activity simultaneously but asynchronously differs from generalized seizures. Focal seizures can migrate from one region to another.

Focal tonic seizures: These are defined by brief but sustained asymmetrical posturing of the trunk or limbs, or tonic deviation of the eyes. In focal tonic seizures, focal seizure activity is almost observed on the EEG. Tonic seizures are the typical seizure form in many neonatal epilepsy syndromes like KCNQ2 developmental and epileptic encephalopathy [15].

Myoclonic seizures: Focal myoclonic movements appear in the form of rapid isolated contractions in the face, a proximal or distal extremity, trunk, or diaphragm. During generalized myoclonic seizures, synchronized contractions occur in both the arms and legs. Myoclonic seizures are characterized by their short duration, absence of slow phase, and selective involvement of flexor muscle groups. Furthermore, certain myoclonic seizures can be triggered by stimulation. Some myoclonic seizures originate from the cortical level, while others arise from more caudal regions such as brainstem or spinal cord. Consequently, pathological EEG findings are observed in some cases, whereas they are absent in others.

Epileptic spasms: It is rarely seen in neonatal period. Truncal muscles and extremities are included. Epileptic spasms can be categorized as flexor, extensor, or mixed type involving both flexor and extensor movements. The neonate's body position at the time of the seizure can affect the clinical appearance of the events. An epileptic spasm begins with a brief muscle contraction and then continues with a phase of muscle relaxation.

Clustered seizures are typically for epileptic spasms and most often observed when the neonate awakens from sleep. A diffuse, high-voltage, slow-wave transient, or a generalized reduction in voltage can be detected on EEG.

Sequential seizures: This type of seizure is frequently seen in neonatal genetic epilepsy syndromes. There is no single type of seizure here, and as the name suggests, there are sequential seizures that vary from one type to another.

2.1 Non-seizure events

Oral, buccal, or lingual movements, swimming, and bicycling movements are motor automatisms in newborns that can be mistaken for neonatal seizures. These movements can be suppressed by restraint or repositioning, and there is no postictal period [16]. Motor automatisms were referred to "subtle seizures" in the past. There are no EEG findings in motor automatisms. Motor automatisms are sometimes associated with electroclinical seizures, but most are nonseizure events. However, in cases of suspected acute brain injury, stereotypic attacks should be evaluated with EEG to determine whether they are seizures.

Myoclonus during the precursor of rapid eye movement [REM] sleep is a normal physiologic condition in neonates. Myoclonus can manifest during periods of quiet or non-REM sleep, and this phenomenon is often termed benign neonatal myoclonus [17]. It is important to distinguish this phenomenon from neonatal seizures, and in healthy newborn, myoclonus typically ceases when the infant wakes up and occurs only during sleep.

Events such as jitteriness and tremulousness can be confused with seizures. These non-seizures events can be suppressed by restraint, and the newborn seems to be in good health.

3. Diagnosis

Neonatal seizures can be diagnosed using an EEG. In the past, only clinical findings were enough for the diagnosis of seizures, and it was named clinical seizures. However, recent EEG studies have demonstrated that electrographic seizures can occur without any noticeable symptoms. Murray et al. and Malone et al. observations reported that when high-risk infants undergo EEG monitoring, there is a significant occurrence of both false positive and false negative clinical diagnosis [18, 19].

The International League Against Epilepsy (ILAE) defined the neonatal seizures an electrographic event defined by sudden, repetitive, evolving stereotyped waveforms with a distinct onset and offset. The duration is not specifically defined, but it must be sufficient to demonstrate changes in frequency and morphology of the discharges and long enough to clearly identify the onset, evolution, and resolution of an abnormal discharge [11].

Multi-channel video continuous EEG (cEEG) monitoring is the gold standard for neonatal seizure diagnosis [20]. If video EEG is not available, serial routine-length EEG or amplitude-integrated EEG (aEEG) with 1- or 2-channel EEG can be useful for demonstrating atypical discharges. The drawbacks of aEEG include the possibility of false positives due to spontaneous movements of the newborn, and the fact that only 30% of seizures detected by conventional EEG is identified by aEEG [21].

4. Etiological evaluation

Gathering a comprehensive history is essential to determine etiology when assessing newborns with seizures. For example, a condition in the pregnancy and birth history can provide us with clues about congenital infection or perinatal asphyxia. The characteristics of other individuals in the family should be examined for familial epileptic syndromes and early unexplained death or inborn errors of metabolism in siblings should also be investigated.

The physical examination findings are crucial for the etiological assessment. The examination should include vital signs, measurement of head size, facial dysmorphologies and somatic abnormalities, and any potential indicators of infection. For example, an atypical facial appearance can guide us towards some genetic syndromes, central nervous system malformations and metabolic diseases. An abnormal odor in sweat or urine can provide a clue towards the diagnosis of a metabolic diseases. Birthmarks such as hemangiomas and skin spots (café au lait spots) are significant signs for neurocutaneous syndromes. The neurological examination should not be overlooked; head circumference, newborn reflexes, the infant's state of mental status and alertness, and any abnormalities in spontaneous movements or muscle tone should be assessed.

Following the anamnesis and physical examination, laboratory tests should promptly be conducted to check serum glucose, calcium, magnesium, and electrolyte levels for rapidly correctable metabolic disorders.

If infection is suspected, blood count, acute phase reactants, and blood culture should be drawn. A lumbar puncture is performed, and after obtaining samples for investigation and culture, initiate appropriate antibiotics, and if necessary, antiviral treatment until meningitis is ruled out.

Initial tests for newborns suspected of having inherited metabolic diseases include; analysis of blood gas, lactate, serum amino acids, urine organic acids, and a tandem acylcarnitine profile.

In newborn experiencing seizures, magnetic resonance imaging (MRI) is the gold standard imaging techniques [22]. MRI is highly valuable for detecting hypoxemic-ischemic encephalopathy, intracranial hemorrhage, ischemic stroke, and brain malformations. For newborns at risk of arterial ischemic stroke, venous sinus thrombosis, or vascular malformations, additional MR angiography or venography can be performed.

Transfontanel ultrasonography (US) should be performed in emergency cases where MRI is not immediately available or clinically unstable newborn. It has high specificity and sensitivity in detecting hydrocephalus and demonstrating intracranial hemorrhage.

Computed tomography (CT) should be avoided in newborns due to the radiation it emits and its inability to provide sufficient information about brain tissue [20].

Genetic testing may be considered in newborns with no etiological causes and suspected epilepsy syndrome.

5. Management of neonatal seizures

In the management of neonatal seizures, the initial steps involve controlling the newborn's airway, breathing, and circulation. Followed by first intervention, fast check-up for some metabolic disturbances such as hypoglycemia, hypocalcemia, and hypomagnesemia. If hypoglycemia is detected, immediately 10% glucose solution should be given intravenously at 2 mL/kg. Then, a maintenance glucose infusion can be given. If a seizure due to hypocalcemia is observed, the newborn should be given 100 mg/kg of 10% calcium gluconate via intravenous infusion. The newborn with hypomagnesemia, 125 mg/kg 50% magnesium sulfate should be administered intramuscularly. In a newborn diagnosed with meningitis or encephalitis, appropriate antibiotic and antiviral treatment should be initiated promptly at suitable doses.

In cases when no cause for the newborn's seizure is identified, initiating antiseizure treatment should be considered. Currently, it is recommended to treat both electro-clinical and only electrographic seizures [11]. Continuous EEG (cEEG) monitoring is very important because abnormal movements of newborns are not seizures, and we cannot identify subclinic electrographic seizures. cEEG protects infants from unnecessary medication and ensures that newborns with subclinic seizures receive appropriate treatment.

6. Antiseizure medications

According to the 2023 guidelines published by the International League Against Epilepsy (ILAE), antiseizure medication protocols have been established [23].

Phenobarbital is still the first choice of initial antiseizure medication therapy drug for infants. It can be used most of seizures with different etiologies. Here are some of the examples:

- Hypoxic-ischemic encephalopathy (HIE)
- Arterial ischemic stroke, intracranial hemorrhage
- Central nervous system (CNS) infection
- Seizures with unknown cause

Phenobarbital is a long-acting barbiturate derivative that exerts its effect by reducing the sensitivity of GABA α receptors. The loading dose of phenobarbital is 20 mg/kg and administered intravenously (IV) infusion. The maintenance dose is 4 to 6 mg/kg per day in two divided doses. If seizures persist after the loading dose, second or third of 10 to 20 mg/kg should be given 1 hour after the first loading dose. Maximum daily dose is 50 mg/kg for phenobarbital.

Phenytoin/fosphenytoin is a sodium channel blocker and first-line antiseizure medication for neonates with a family history of epilepsy due to a channelopathy. The initial dose is 15 to 20 mg/kg, via intravenous, at a rate of 3 mg/kg/per minute, followed by a maintenance dose of 4 to 8 mg/kg/day administered 12 hours later.

Levetiracetam: It is the preferred second-line antiseizure medication for neonates with cardiac disorders [23]. The loading dose of levetiracetam is recommended 60 mg/kg intravenously, followed by a maintenance dose of 60 mg/kg/day divided into three doses [24]. According to NEOLEV2 study, loading levetiracetam is ineffective to provide immediate seizure control as first- or second-line medication for neonates who have persistent seizures after phenobarbital administration [25].

Midazolam: It is an antiseizure medication and a form of benzodiazepine group. Also, it can be used for pre-intubation and sedation in neonates. Midazolam is typically administered as a bolus of 150 mcg/kg followed by continuous infusion starting at 1 mcg/kg/mn. Due to the potential for midazolam to depress the respiratory system, it is important to closely monitor these newborns for respiratory and cardiovascular function.

Lidocaine: This is a class 1b anti-arrhythmic agent that exerts its antiseizure effect by blocking voltage-gated sodium channels. It can be used for neonatal seizures in selected patients. In cases of status epilepticus verified in EEG, even with the maximum phenobarbital dose, intravenous lidocaine infusion can be considered as a second-line medication, if there are no contraindications to its use and pretreatment with fosphenytoin/phenytoin. Lidocaine is contraindicated newborns with congenital heart disease. Initial bolus dose of lidocaine is (2 mg/kg over 10 minutes), continued with an infusion of 7 mg/kg for 4 hours. After 4 hours, decrease the dose by %50 every 12 hours. Lidocaine itself is also a proarrhythmic agent, so its use is not recommended over than 48 hours.

6.1 Treatment-resistant seizures

Sometimes seizures may persist despite multiple antiseizure medications. In cases, who do not respond to conventional antiseizure therapy and unknown etiology, administration of pyridoxine and pyridoxal-5-phosphate should be considered. Pyridoxine is administrated 100 mg intravenous injections and can be repeated every 5 to 15 minutes up to a maximum of 500 mg. This case should be monitored with continuous EEG monitoring. If the patient do not respond to therapy again, folinic acid 2.5 mg should be given intravenously.

Biotinidase deficiency may cause refractory neonatal seizures that are responsive to oral biotin supplementation.

7. Conclusion

Neonatal seizures are one of the most common emergency neurological diseases in the neonatal period. The prognosis of neonatal seizures is heavily influenced by the primary etiology. Other factors that can affect the prognosis are the gestational age and birth weight of newborn, APGAR score, postnatal age of infant when the seizure starts, and the type and duration of seizures. Today, we still do not know which seizures cause brain damage and which do not. But we know continuous EEG monitoring is essential for starting therapy and determining when to discontinue treatment in these infants. It seems that phenobarbital remains the first-line antiseizure drug in treatment.

Author details

Duygu Acar
Neonatal İntensive Care Unit, Gaziosmanpasa Research and Training Hospital, Istanbul, Turkey

*Address all correspondence to: dbesnili@hotmail.com

References

[1] Lanska MJ, Lanska DJ, Baumann RJ, Kryscio RJ. A population-based study of neonatal seizures in Fayette County, Kentucky. Neurology. 1995;**45**:724

[2] Ronen GM, Penney S, Andrews W. The epidemiology of clinical neonatal seizures in Newfoundland: A population-based study. The Journal of Pediatrics. 1999;**134**:71

[3] Saliba RM, Annegers JF, Waller DK, et al. Incidence of neonatal seizures in Harris County, Texas, 1992-1994. American Journal of Epidemiology. 1999;**150**:763

[4] Scher MS, Aso K, Beggarly ME, et al. Electrographic seizures in preterm and full-term neonates: Clinical correlates, associated brain lesions, and risk for neurologic sequelae. Pediatrics. 1993;**91**:128

[5] Glass HC, Pham TN, Danielsen B, et al. Antenatal and intrapartum risk factors for seizures in term newborns: A population-based study, California 1998-2002. The Journal of Pediatrics. 2009;**154**:24

[6] Pisani F, Facini C, Bianchi E, et al. Incidence of neonatal seizures, perinatal risk factors for epilepsy and mortality after neonatal seizures in the province of Parma, Italy. Epilepsia. 2018;**59**:1764

[7] Co JP, Elia M, Engel J Jr, et al. Proposal of an algorithm for diagnosis and treatment of neonatal seizures in developing countries. Epilepsia. 2007;**48**:1158

[8] Mizrahi E, Watanabe K. Symptomatic neonatal seizures. In: Roger J, Bureau M, Dravet C, Genton P, Tassinari CA, Wolf P, editors. Epileptic Syndromes in Infancy, Childhood and Adolescence. 3. London: John Libbey & Co Ltd; 2002. pp. 15-31

[9] Chapman KE, Mizrahi EM, Clancy RR. Neonatal seizures. In: Wyllie A, Cascino GD, Gidal BE, Goodkin HP, editors. Wyllie's Treatment of Epilepsy: Principles and Practice. 5th ed. Philadelphia: Lippincott, Williams & Wilkens; 2011. p. 405

[10] Glass HC, Shellhaas RA, Wusthoff CJ, et al. Contemporary profile of seizures in neonates: A prospective cohort study. The Journal of Pediatrics. 2016;**174**:98

[11] Pressler RM, Cilio MR, Mizrahi EM, et al. The ILAE classification of seizures and the epilepsies: Modification for seizures in the neonate. Position paper by the ILAE task force on neonatal seizures. Epilepsia. 2021;**62**:615

[12] Shellhaas RA, Wusthoff CJ, Tsuchida TN, et al. Profile of neonatal epilepsies: Characteristics of a prospective US cohort. Neurology. 2017;**89**:893

[13] Wusthoff CJ, Dlugos DJ, Gutierrez-Colina A, et al. Electrographic seizures during therapeutic hypothermia for neonatal hypoxic-ischemic encephalopathy. Journal of Child Neurology. 2011;**26**:724

[14] Lloyd RO, O'Toole JM, Pavlidis E, et al. Electrographic seizures during the early postnatal period in preterm infants. The Journal of Pediatrics. 2017;**187**:18

[15] Zuberi SM, Wirrell E, Yozawitz E, et al. ILAE classification and definition of epilepsy syndromes with onset in neonates and infants: Position statement by the ILAE task force on nosology and definitions. Epilepsia. 2022;**63**:1349

[16] Mizrahi EM, Kellaway P. Characterization and classification of neonatal seizures. Neurology. 1987;**37**:1837

[17] Di Capua M, Fusco L, Ricci S, Vigevano F. Benign neonatal sleep myoclonus: Clinical features and video-polygraphic recordings. Movement Disorders. 1993;**8**:191

[18] Murray DM, Boylan GB, Ali I, et al. Defining the gap between electrographic seizure burden, clinical expression and staff recognition of neonatal seizures. Archives of Disease in Childhood. Fetal and Neonatal Edition. 2008;**93**:F187

[19] Malone A, Ryan CA, Fitzgerald A, et al. Interobserver agreement in neonatal seizure identification. Epilepsia. 2009;**50**:2097

[20] Shellhaas RA, Chang T, Tsuchida T, et al. The American clinical neurophysiology Society's guideline on continuous electroencephalography monitoring in neonates. Journal of Clinical Neurophysiology. 2011;**28**:611

[21] Hellström-Westas L. Amplitude-integrated electroencephalography for seizure detection in newborn infants. Seminars in Fetal & Neonatal Medicine. 2018;**23**:175-182

[22] Glass HC, Bonifacio SL, Sullivan J, Rogers E, Ferriero DM, Goldstein R, et al. Magnetic resonance imaging and ultrasound injury in preterm infants with seizures. Journal of Child Neurology. 2009;**24**:1105-1111

[23] Pressler RM, Abend NS, Auvin S, et al. Treatment of seizures in the neonate: Guidelines and consensus-based recommendations-special report from the ILAE task force on neonatal seizures. Epilepsia. 2023;**64**:2550

[24] Sharpe CM, Capparelli EV, Mower A, et al. A seven-day study of the pharmacokinetics of intravenous levetiracetam in neonates: Marked changes in pharmacokinetics occur during the first week of life. Pediatric Research. 2012;**72**:43

[25] Sharpe C, Reiner GE, Davis SL, et al. Levetiracetam versus phenobarbital for neonatal seizures: A randomized controlled trial. Pediatrics. 2020;**145**(6)

Chapter 7

Hypoxic Ischemic Encephalopathy, Therapeutic Hypothermia, and Novel Combinations

Erhan Aygün and Seda Yilmaz Semerci

Abstract

Hypoxic-ischemic encephalopathy is a serious entity that leads to impaired neurological function and can result in death or long-term developmental challenges. Early recognition and intervention, particularly through therapeutic hypothermia initiated within 6 hours after birth, are critical. Hypothermia is indicated in cases with signs of perinatal asphyxia and moderate-to-severe neurological symptoms, and is shown to reduce both mortality and developmental disabilities. Due to the limited effectiveness of therapeutic hypothermia in some instances, there is an urgent need for novel combination therapies to maximize the benefit. Adjunctive treatments, including darbepoetin and allopurinol, along with emerging agents like stem cell therapy and sovateltide, are designed to enhance neuroprotection. However, their effects are still limited. Therefore, a comprehensive understanding of the pathophysiology is essential for developing effective interventions that can improve neonatal outcomes and address long-term neurological issues. Future studies should focus on integrated strategies that address both the immediate and lasting effects of brain injury.

Keywords: hypoxic ischemic encephalopathy, neuroprotection, novel therapeutic agents, therapeutic hypothermia, newborn

1. Introduction

Neonatal encephalopathy (NE) is a clinical syndrome characterized by changes in neurological function, evidenced by difficulties in initiating and maintaining respiration at birth or shortly thereafter, decreased levels of consciousness, suppressed muscle tone and reflexes, disturbances in cranial nerve function, and possible seizure activity [1]. Neonatal encephalopathy is a general term that describes a syndrome that can occur due to various causes, including brain malformations, intracranial hemorrhage, stroke, metabolic disorders, genetic disorders, infections, toxin exposure, and hypoxic-ischemic encephalopathy (HIE). Neonatal encephalopathy occurs in approximately 3 out of every 1000 live births, and about 50% of these cases are attributed to HIE [2]. Timely recognition and prevention of HIE, which can lead to death or severe neurodevelopmental disorders (cognitive impairment, cerebral palsy, seizures, and neurosensory deficits), is crucial in increasing the survival of newborns without sequelae [3].

2. HIE pathogenesis and therapeutic hypothermia

Severe hypoxia-ischemia that can damage the brain leads to a critical decrease in the transport of oxygen and glucose to the brain, triggering a series of early and later developing pathological events [4]. The initial effect of hypoxic-ischemic conditions is a decrease in levels of high-energy phosphorylation compounds including adenosine triphosphate (ATP) and phosphocreatine (PCr), leading to primary energy deficiency. Primary energy deficiency triggers numerous cellular events that depend on energy [5]. If resuscitation is performed in a timely and successful manner, ATP and PCr levels can be achieved again, initiating a 'latent phase' that lasts approximately 6 hours. In this phase, mitochondrial dysfunction can occur, serving as a key factor in determining whether subsequent damage develops [6]. Hence, impaired mitochondrial function can be a trigger for the second energy deficiency period, which occurs 6–12 hours after hypoxia-ischemia [7].

Secondary energy deficiency presents with ongoing excitotoxicity and free radical damage, accompanied by different pathogenic processes compared to primary energy deficiency (inflammation, accelerated apoptosis, loss of synaptic connections). This second phase can last from hours to days and is followed by the development of a 'tertiary phase' characterized by the clearance of necrotic and apoptotic tissues, scar formation (gliosis), and a reduction in brain volume (global or regional). At the same time, tissue repair processes, including stem cell proliferation, angiogenesis, and the re-establishment of synaptic connections, begin, and these processes can take weeks to months [8, 9].

The neuroprotection provided by hypothermia positively modifies processes of primary and secondary energy deficiency and the latent phase by affecting multiple mechanisms rather than a single pathway [10]. Hypothermia has several effects on the body, including reducing brain energy consumption, aligning blood flow with metabolic needs, decreasing the release of excitatory neurotransmitters, suppressing the production of reactive oxygen species, inhibiting inflammation, and slowing the process of apoptotic cell death. However, hypothermia is not effective in supporting neurologic tissue amelioration.

Experimental studies showed that hypothermia is most effective when initiated within the first 6 hours after hypoxia-ischemia. Based on these findings, the latent phase is considered a 'therapeutic window' for initiating treatment, providing an opportunity to reduce or prevent brain damage [11, 12].

2.1 Criteria for initiating therapeutic hypothermia

In neonates with HIE, significant risk factors related to the maternal antepartum period, including chronic hypertension, diabetes, or antepartum bleeding, are common. Besides, the frequency of intrapartum complications is relatively high, and these events are part of the pathways that lead to the development of acute fetal hypoxia-ischemia [13]. Most intrapartum complications occur unexpectedly, and some are considered sentinel events.

However, according to the American College of Obstetricians and Gynecologists (ACOG) Neonatal Encephalopathy Task Force report, there is no diagnostic test that indicates the timing for HIE [1].

To evaluate the impact of acute peripartum or intrapartum hypoxia-ischemia on a newborn with encephalopathy, several factors should be considered. These include a significant event during or before delivery, abnormal fetal heart rate patterns, low Apgar scores, signs of fetal acidosis, encephalopathy, seizures in the newborn, EEG evidence of encephalopathy, multisystem organ dysfunction, MRI findings, placental issues, and the exclusion of other potential causes of encephalopathy. Since the symptoms of HIE can gradually emerge over hours to days following birth, serial neurological examinations, follow-up of EEG findings, assessment of organ dysfunction outside the central nervous system, and MRI findings are necessary. Therefore, the presence of multiple criteria together strengthens the HIE diagnosis and stresses the association between peripartum events and neurodevelopmental outcomes in childhood.

In general, the inclusion criteria focus on clinical or biochemical evidence of impaired placental gas exchange, followed by findings of moderate or severe encephalopathy according to modified Sarnat stages [14–18]. The presence of encephalopathy is a vital sign that confirms the biological effects of placental gas exchange.

Inclusion Criteria for Therapeutic Hypothermia:

1. *Gestational age and birth weight*

   ≥ 36 weeks of gestation, birth weight > 1800 grams

2. *Time to onset of hypothermia after birth: First 6 hours*

3. *Signs of disturbance in placental gas exchange (one or more of the following)*

   - Low Apgar scores (< 5)
   - Need for resuscitation
   - Fetal acidosis (e.g., low pH or base excess)

4. *Neurological examination:*

   Moderate or severe encephalopathy (according to modified Sarnat staging) (31–34).

5. *Electrophysiological evidence:*

Encephalopathy findings on amplitude-integrated EEG (aEEG) or EEG (31–33).

Exclusion criteria:

Patients with mild encephalopathy were not included in any study.

Newborns diagnosed with brain malformation, and metabolic or neuromuscular disease.

Infants with positive blood cultures.

Therapeutic hypothermia should start within the first 6-hour latent period during which the best response to treatment is obtained. Although there is no definitive diagnostic test for HIE, the above criteria aim to identify high-risk infants based on clinical, biochemical, and neurophysiological findings.

2.2 The effectiveness of therapeutic hypothermia for HIE

Therapeutic hypothermia is the treatment of choice and evidence-based therapy for HIE—this evidence is based on the data from a meta-analysis on hypothermia for HIE [19]. Standard practices regarding therapeutic hypothermia included a step-by-step inclusion process, randomization into cooling or standard care groups, a 72-hour cooling period, and rewarming at a rate of 0.5°C per hour. Two cooling methods can be employed: whole-body cooling (targeting 33.5°C) and head cooling with lighter body cooling (targeting 34.5°C). Severe disabilities from HIE included cerebral palsy, significant developmental delays, blindness, and hearing loss.

The effectiveness of hypothermia is found to be consistent between both cooling methods, although some rare adverse effects were reported, including bradycardia and thrombocytopenia. Follow-up studies at 6–7 years revealed lower mortality rates in the cooling group compared to standard care, but no significant differences in rates of cerebral palsy or severe disabilities. Notably, children treated with hypothermia demonstrated better educational and behavioral outcomes than those receiving standard care, but their long-term educational needs remained significant [20]. Therefore, scientific efforts focused on developing new agents or combination therapies to improve the outcomes for infants affected by HIE.

2.2.1 Deeper and longer cooling

In a study conducted between 2010 and 2013, researchers attempted to reduce mortality and its sequelae by using deeper (32.5°C) and longer cooling (120 hours) methods [21]. However, this approach did not yield any additional benefits compared to standard treatment.

In a randomized controlled trial conducted in India, Sri Lanka, and Bangladesh, researchers explored the effects of hypothermia on newborns with moderate or severe encephalopathy compared to standard care [22]. The hypothermia treatment was initiated within 6 hours after birth and continued for 72 hours, while infants in the control group received only supportive intensive care. The results indicated that hypothermia treatment did not reduce mortality or disability rates; in fact, the mortality rate increased. These findings imply that brain damage may begin before birth, suggesting that the optimal window for effective hypothermia treatment could be compromised. Besides, the quality of birth practices emerged as a critical factor, particularly given the low rates of emergency Cesarean sections. The discrepancies between this study and those conducted in the United States underscore the need for future research involving larger participant cohorts.

2.3 How is hypothermia treatment applied?

There are two methods for therapeutic hypothermia. One of these methods is the use of a cooling helmet (cap) through which cold water circulates, allowing the body temperature to be lowered to 34.5°C. The cooling cap minimizes the drop in body temperature required for cooling deep brain regions.

The other approach is to cool the brain by lowering body temperature. Nowadays, the cooling cap method is largely abandoned, and whole-body cooling is the most commonly used method.

The newborn infant is placed on a cooling blanket, and the body temperature is reduced to 33.5°C (acceptable range: 33.0–34) to ensure a decrease in brain temperature as well.

The core body temperature is usually monitored using a probe placed in the lower third of the esophagus or the rectum [23].

2.4 The long-term effects of HIE and hypothermia on families

Therapeutic hypothermia and HIE diagnosis are situation that creates intense stress for families. The family is faced with witnessing emergency interventions related to their baby's health issues, instead of the expected healthy birth. This process can negatively affect the mother-baby bonding and increase the risk of postpartum depression, anxiety, and post-traumatic stress disorder in mothers [24, 25].

The adverse effects of HIE and hypothermia on the family begin with the loss of the mother-baby bonding process at birth; this situation includes the mother being separated from her baby immediately, the inability to provide skin-to-skin contact, and the inability to start breastfeeding. Although mothers of neonates with acute illness experience a similar separation, the effects of HIE on the maternal experience are further amplified due to the uncertainty of the prognosis during the hospitalization period. Interventions focusing on communication, the integration of the parents' involvement in the caregiving process, mental health, and social support are recommended, based on the principles of trauma-informed care, to address the trauma associated with HIE [25, 26]. During hypothermia treatment, families should be encouraged to be by their baby's side. A limited number of studies suggest that this practice can be possible and beneficial under certain conditions [27, 28].

3. Novel combination therapies

3.1 Erythropoietin and darbepoetin

Erythropoietin (EPO) is a hormone necessary for the production of red blood cells and is primarily produced by the kidneys. Cellular hypoxia responses regulate EPO production and are generally inversely proportional to oxygen levels; its production increases in hypoxic conditions [29]. In a hypoxic condition, EPO gene expression increases through the binding of HIF-2α to the hypoxic response element in the EPO gene [30]. EPO stimulates the production of red blood cells by interacting with EPO receptors (EPOR) on erythroid progenitor cells and some erythroid non-progenitor cells [31]. However, EPO has inhibitory effects on adipogenesis and osteogenesis. The clinical data indicate that adding EPO to hypothermia does not provide a significant benefit in the treatment of HIE, despite having neuroprotective potential. Furthermore, adverse effects such as thrombosis and intracranial hemorrhage have been reported for EPO.

Darbepoetin is a more stable analogue of EPO, with a longer half-life and higher biological activity, but it has a lower affinity for EPOR [32]. Although the benefits of using darbepoetin along with therapeutic hypothermia were demonstrated, further research is needed for its use in routine clinical practice [33].

3.2 Topiramate

In newborns diagnosed with HIE, the combined use of topiramate and hypothermia treatment did not show a significant difference in mortality and seizure activity compared to placebo administered alongside hypothermia.

When evaluated at a higher dose (10 mg/kg for 3 days), it is confirmed that topiramate is safe and well-tolerated when administered with hypothermia. However, the neuroprotective effects described in animal models cannot be validated in newborns with hypoxic-ischemic encephalopathy (HIE). The combined application of topiramate and hypothermia did not reduce mortality, brain damage, sensory disorders, or the frequency of neurodevelopmental issues assessed by motor and cognitive scores. The effects of topiramate on molecular damage markers in newborns with HIE have not been sufficiently studied yet; therefore, appropriate evaluations are needed to validate the findings reported in animal models [31, 34].

3.3 Glucocorticoids

Glucocorticoids are shown to enhance neuroprotection after hypoxic-ischemic (HI) damage when applied to the neonatal brain, in addition to their homeostatic functions such as blood pressure regulation, immune system modulation, and metabolism [35]. Notably, hydrocortisone was tested in a phase II/III study, where it was found that the group administered low doses had a significant increase in blood pressure compared to the placebo group [36]. The study also revealed that hydrocortisone reduces inotropic requirements during hypothermia treatment. However, current treatment methods do not effectively repair neuronal damage caused by hypoxic-ischemic encephalopathy (HIE). They are only beneficial in some instances, underscoring the need for new treatment options and the prevention of neuronal damage.

3.4 Melatonin

Melatonin is a neurohormone with antioxidant and anti-inflammatory properties. In preclinical models, it has been demonstrated to reduce apoptosis in brain tissue and mitigate oxidative stress when combined with hypothermia. Although some clinical studies have indicated that melatonin may have the potential to improve neurodevelopmental outcomes in HIE, further studies are needed to provide definitive recommendations [37].

3.5 Caffeine

Caffeine is a commonly used natural stimulant that acts on adenosine receptors and belongs to the methylxanthine class. In animal models, caffeine reduces damage to brain white matter [38]. In preterm newborns, caffeine is found to be effective in reducing acute kidney injury (AKI) [39]. However, the safety and efficacy of caffeine have not yet been studied in newborns with HIE who undergo therapeutic hypothermia.

3.6 Citicoline

Citicoline is an exogenous formulation of cytidine 5′-diphosphocholine that offers neuroprotective effects by reducing glutamate accumulation, promoting the repair of damaged cell membranes, and preventing oxidative stress [40]. In the context of HIE, it holds promise as a potential neuroprotective agent.

A small-scale randomized study demonstrated that citicoline improves short-term outcomes [41]. Currently, a Phase I study in Pakistan is investigating the effects of a combination of therapeutic hypothermia and citicoline. Targeting multiple cellular mechanisms at different time points is thought to provide greater neuroprotection compared to using a single agent [8].

3.7 Metformin

Metformin is a common biguanide used in the treatment of type 2 diabetes, with a high ability to cross the blood-brain barrier. It is being evaluated as a potential drug candidate for central nervous system diseases due to its antioxidant, anti-inflammatory, anti-apoptotic, and antitumor properties [42]. Experimental studies have revealed that metformin exhibits neuroprotective effects in spinal cord injuries and cerebral ischemia/reperfusion damage, as well as positive effects such as supporting neurogenesis, maintaining blood-brain barrier (BBB) integrity, and promoting remyelination in newborns [43, 44]. Metformin is thought to be supportive for remyelination after white matter injury in newborns [45]. However, its effects on neonatal brain damage related to hypoxic-ischemic events remain unclear, and further research is needed on its neuroprotective potential.

3.8 Allopurinol

Allopurinol prevents the formation of superoxide radicals following hypoxic-ischemic brain damage by inhibiting xanthine oxidase.

Kaandorp and colleagues found that in infants with HIE who were administered allopurinol within the first 4 hours after birth, neurodevelopmental outcomes were better between the ages of 4 and 8 [46]. Gunes and his colleagues reported that in newborns who received allopurinol within the first 2 hours after birth, the 12-month neurodevelopmental outcomes were better [47].

However, both studies were conducted before the widespread use of therapeutic hypothermia, and therefore do not reflect the use of allopurinol as an adjunctive treatment alongside hypothermia. The phase III ALBINO study will evaluate the effects of allopurinol administered in conjunction with therapeutic hypothermia on the 24-month mortality rate and severe neurodevelopmental disorders [48].

3.9 Stem cells

Multipotent stem cells are special cells that can self-renew and differentiate into various cell types specific to different tissues. Several types of stem cells demonstrate therapeutic potential for treating hypoxic-ischemic injury, including mesenchymal stem cells (MSCs), inducible pluripotent stem cells (iPSCs), mononuclear cells, neural stem cells, oligodendrocyte progenitor cells, hematopoietic stem cells, and endothelial cells [49].

These cells have positive effects at both the cellular and functional levels. Stem cells contribute to better functional outcomes after damage by creating a suitable microenvironment for tissue regeneration [50]. While stem cell applications showed positive effects in preclinical and clinical studies following perinatal hypoxic-ischemic injury, further studies are needed for routine use [51, 52].

3.10 Sovateltide

Sovateltide (IRL-1620 or PMZ-1620) is a synthetic analog of ET-1 and is an agonist that binds with high specificity to endothelin B (ETB) receptors [53]. Numerous studies demonstrated that sovateltide positively alters brain injury recovery by inhibiting apoptosis, reducing oxidative stress, promoting angiogenesis and neurogenesis, and facilitating neuronal repair and regeneration [54, 55]. These effects collectively lead to enhancements in neurological and motor functions. Sovateltide is currently being studied as a 'first-in-class' drug candidate for the treatment of HIE.

Experimental studies revealed an increase in survival rates, a decrease in neurological and motor deficits, a reduction in stroke volume, edema, and oxidative stress levels, as well as an increase in hypoxia-related survival factors [56].

Sovateltide is recently approved as a safe, well-tolerated, and effective treatment when initiated within the first 24 hours for patients with acute ischemic stroke in India [57]. In preclinical studies conducted on HIE models, it is shown to reduce oxidative and hypoxic damage, promoting recovery in damaged brain tissue by inducing angiogenesis and neurogenesis. Sovateltide owns multiple effects needed to both stop HIE-related damage and promote neuronal regeneration.

In the future, stem cells and new treatment candidates with multiple mechanisms of action, including sovateltide, allopurinol, and melatonin, could be effective and promising agents as adjuncts to hypothermia in the treatment of HIE.

4. Mitochondria-targeted therapeutic approaches

Intracellular ATP depletion plays a central role in the pathogenesis of HIE, with mitochondria at the heart of the pathological cascade involving oxidative stress, inflammation, and cell death [58]. Therefore, mitochondria-targeted therapies offer a promising adjunct to current therapeutic hypothermia strategies. Mitochondrial therapy encompasses a range of approaches designed to enhance mitochondrial function, either through replacement methods or by strengthening existing mitochondrial activity. Agents such as EPO and MitoSNO are shown to directly preserve mitochondrial function by reducing reactive oxygen species (ROS) production and preventing neuronal chromatin damage [59].

Furthermore, strategies aimed at modulating mitochondrial dynamics (e.g., fusion and fission processes), enhancing mitochondrial biogenesis, and stimulating mitophagy show great potential in restoring cellular energy balance and limiting secondary injury in the neonatal brain [60]. Through these approaches, mitochondrial proton leak can be minimized, ATP synthesis can be supported, and inflammatory cascades can be attenuated. While preclinical data primarily support these strategies, they represent a growing framework for addressing both acute energy failure and long-term neurodevelopmental deficits in infants with HIE.

5. Conclusion

Novel therapies for HIE in newborns are a challenging but rapidly evolving field. Finding effective treatments requires a comprehensive understanding of the disease's pathophysiology, rigorous preclinical testing, well-designed clinical trials, and an approach focused on long-term clinical outcomes. The goal is to improve long-term outcomes and enhance the quality of life for infants with HIE. To date, in clinical studies on HIE, no adjunctive therapy has provided additional benefits beyond hypothermia. A common limitation of these adjuncts is that while they can control secondary phase events of HIE to limit brain damage, they do not repair neuronal injury. Therefore, there is a need for the development and evaluation of new therapies or adjunctive drugs that support neurogenesis and angiogenesis. These treatments could be effective in both preventing and repairing neuronal damage after HIE.

Conflict of interest

The authors declare no conflict of interest.

Author details

Erhan Aygün[1] and Seda Yilmaz Semerci[2*]

1 University of Health Sciences, Kanuni Sultan Suleyman Training and Research Hospital, Istanbul, Turkiye

2 Istinye University, School of Medicine, Istanbul, Turkiye

*Address all correspondence to: sedayilmazsemerci@gmail.com

References

[1] Executive Summary: Neonatal Encephalopathy and Neurologic Outcome, Second Edition. Report of the American College of Obstetricians and Gynecologists' Task Force on Neonatal Encephalopathy. Obstetrics and Gynecology. 2014;**123**:896-901

[2] Kurinczuk JJ, White-Koning M, Badawi N. Epidemiology of neonatal encephalopathy and hypoxic-ischaemic encephalopathy. Early Human Development. 2010;**86**:329-338

[3] Natarajan G, McDonald SA, Shankaran S, et al. Prediction of neurodevelopmental outcomes at 18 to 22 months using the numerical Sarnat score compared with modified Sarnat staging in infants with moderate to severe hypoxic-ischemic encephalopathy. The Journal of Pediatrics. 2025;**281**:114522

[4] Davidson JO, Gonzalez F, Gressens P, et al. Update on mechanisms of the pathophysiology of neonatal encephalopathy. Seminars in Fetal and Neonatal Medicine. 2021;**26**:101267

[5] Kratimenos P, Koutroulis I, Jain A, et al. Effect of concurrent Src kinase inhibition with short-duration hypothermia on Ca²⁺/calmodulin kinase IV activity and neuropathology after hypoxia-ischemia in the newborn swine brain. Neonatology. 2018;**113**:37-43

[6] Samaiya PK, Krishnamurthy S, Kumar A. Mitochondrial dysfunction in perinatal asphyxia: Role in pathogenesis and potential therapeutic interventions. Molecular and Cellular Biochemistry. 2021;**476**:4421-4434

[7] Mitra S, Bale G, Mathieson S, et al. Changes in cerebral oxidative metabolism during neonatal seizures following hypoxic-ischemic brain injury. Frontiers in Pediatrics. 2016;**4**:83

[8] Chan NH, Hawkins CC, Rodrigues BV, et al. Neuroprotection for neonatal hypoxic–ischemic encephalopathy: A review of novel therapies evaluated in clinical studies. Developmental Medicine and Child Neurology. 2025;**67**:591-599

[9] Babbo CC-R, Mellet J, van Rensburg J, et al. Neonatal encephalopathy due to suspected hypoxic ischemic encephalopathy: Pathophysiology, current, and emerging treatments. World Journal of Pediatrics. 2024;**20**:1105-1114

[10] Yenari MA, Han HS. Neuroprotective mechanisms of hypothermia in brain ischaemia. Nature Reviews. Neuroscience. 2012;**13**:267-278

[11] Gunn AJ, Gunn TR, de Haan HH, et al. Dramatic neuronal rescue with prolonged selective head cooling after ischemia in fetal lambs. The Journal of Clinical Investigation. 1997;**99**:248-256

[12] Gunn AJ, Bennet L, Gunning MI, et al. Cerebral hypothermia is not neuroprotective when started after postischemic seizures in fetal sheep. Pediatric Research. 1999;**46**:274-280

[13] Roto S, Nupponen I, Kalliala I, et al. Risk factors for neonatal hypoxic ischemic encephalopathy and therapeutic hypothermia: A matched case-control study. BMC Pregnancy and Childbirth. 2024;**24**:421

[14] Shankaran S, Laptook AR, Ehrenkranz RA, et al. Whole-body hypothermia for neonates with hypoxic-ischemic encephalopathy.

The New England Journal of Medicine. 2005;**353**:1574-1584

[15] Gluckman PD, Wyatt JS, Azzopardi D, et al. Selective head cooling with mild systemic hypothermia after neonatal encephalopathy: Multicentre randomised trial. Lancet. 2005;**365**:663-670

[16] Azzopardi DV, Strohm B, Edwards AD, et al. Moderate hypothermia to treat perinatal asphyxial encephalopathy. The New England Journal of Medicine. 2009;**361**:1349-1358

[17] Simbruner G, Mittal RA, Rohlmann F, et al. Systemic hypothermia after neonatal encephalopathy: Outcomes of neo.nEURO.Network RCT. Pediatrics. 2010;**126**:e771-e778

[18] Jacobs SE, Morley CJ, Inder TE, et al. Whole-body hypothermia for term and near-term newborns with hypoxic-ischemic encephalopathy: A randomized controlled trial. Archives of Pediatrics and Adolescent Medicine. 2011;**165**:692-700

[19] Jacobs SE, Berg M, Hunt R, et al. Cooling for newborns with hypoxic ischaemic encephalopathy. Cochrane Database of Systematic Reviews. 2013;**2013**:CD003311

[20] van Oldenmark BO, van Steenis A, de Vries LS, et al. Fifteen years of neonatal therapeutic hypothermia: Clinical trends show unchanged post-rewarming outcomes despite reduction in hypoxic-ischemic encephalopathy severity. Neonatology. 2025;**122**(2):191-201

[21] Shankaran S, Laptook AR, Pappas A, et al. Effect of depth and duration of cooling on death or disability at age 18 months among neonates with hypoxic-ischemic encephalopathy: A randomized clinical trial. JAMA. 2017;**318**:57-67

[22] Thayyil S, Pant S, Montaldo P, et al. Hypothermia for moderate or severe neonatal encephalopathy in low-income and middle-income countries (HELIX): A randomised controlled trial in India, Sri Lanka, and Bangladesh. The Lancet Global Health. 2021;**9**:e1273-e1285

[23] Enweronu-Laryea C, Martinello KA, Rose M, et al. Core temperature after birth in babies with neonatal encephalopathy in a sub-Saharan African hospital setting. The Journal of Physiology. 2019;**597**:4013-4024

[24] Laudi A, Peeples E. The relationship between neonatal encephalopathy and maternal postpartum depression. The Journal of Maternal-Fetal and Neonatal Medicine. 2020;**33**:3313-3317

[25] Sagaser A, Pilon B, Goeller A, et al. Parent experience of hypoxic-ischemic encephalopathy and hypothermia: A call for trauma informed care. American Journal of Perinatology. 2024;**41**:586-593

[26] Craig AK, Munoz-Blanco S, Pilon B, et al. Communicating with parents about therapeutic hypothermia and hypoxic ischemic encephalopathy: Integrating a palliative care approach into practice. Clinics in Perinatology. 2024;**51**:711-724

[27] Ingram J, Beasant L, Odd D, et al. Opportunity to bond and a sense of normality': Parent and staff views of cuddling babies undergoing therapeutic hypothermia in neonatal intensive care: 'CoolCuddle'. Health Expectations. 2022;**25**:1384-1392

[28] Beasant L, Chakkarapani E, Horwood J, et al. Embedding the 'CoolCuddle' intervention for infants undergoing therapeutic hypothermia for hypoxic-ischaemic encephalopathy in NICU: An evaluation using normalisation process theory. BMJ Open. 2024;**14**:e088228

[29] Li J, Quan C, He Y-L, et al. Autophagy regulated by the HIF/REDD1/mTORC1 signaling is progressively increased during erythroid differentiation under hypoxia. Frontiers in Cell and Development Biology. 2022;**10**:896893

[30] Suzuki N, Gradin K, Poellinger L, et al. Regulation of hypoxia-inducible gene expression after HIF activation. Experimental Cell Research. 2017;**356**:182-186

[31] Marques KL, Rodrigues V, Balduci CTN, et al. Emerging therapeutic strategies in hypoxic-ischemic encephalopathy: A focus on cognitive outcomes. Frontiers in Pharmacology. 2024;**15**:1347529

[32] Egrie JC, Dwyer E, Browne JK, et al. Darbepoetin alfa has a longer circulating half-life and greater in vivo potency than recombinant human erythropoietin. Experimental Hematology. 2003;**31**:290-299

[33] Molloy EJ, El-Dib M, Soul J, et al. Neuroprotective therapies in the NICU in preterm infants: Present and future (neonatal Neurocritical care series). Pediatric Research. 2024;**95**:1224-1236

[34] Nuñez-Ramiro A, Benavente-Fernández I, Valverde E, et al. Topiramate plus cooling for hypoxic-ischemic encephalopathy: A randomized, controlled, multicenter, double-blinded trial. Neonatology. 2019;**116**:76-84

[35] Concepcion KR, Zhang L. Corticosteroids and perinatal hypoxic-ischemic brain injury. Drug Discovery Today. 2018;**23**:1718-1732

[36] Kovacs K, Szakmar E, Meder U, et al. A randomized controlled study of low-dose hydrocortisone versus placebo in dopamine-treated hypotensive neonates undergoing hypothermia treatment for hypoxic–ischemic encephalopathy. The Journal of Pediatrics. 2019;**211**:13-19.e3

[37] Pluta R, Furmaga-Jabłońska W, Januszewski S, et al. Melatonin: A potential candidate for the treatment of experimental and clinical perinatal asphyxia. Molecules. 2023;**28**:1105

[38] Yang L, Yu X, Zhang Y, et al. Caffeine treatment started before injury reduces hypoxic–ischemic white-matter damage in neonatal rats by regulating phenotypic microglia polarization. Pediatric Research. 2022;**92**:1543-1554

[39] Harer MW, Askenazi DJ, Boohaker LJ, et al. Association between early caffeine citrate administration and risk of acute kidney injury in preterm neonates. JAMA Pediatrics. 2018;**172**:e180322

[40] Jasielski P, Piędel F, Piwek M, et al. Application of citicoline in neurological disorders: A systematic review. Nutrients. 2020;**12**:3113

[41] Salamah A, El Amrousy D, Elsheikh M, et al. Citicoline in hypoxic ischemic encephalopathy in neonates: A randomized controlled trial. Italian Journal of Pediatrics. 2023;**49**:55

[42] Mei J, Li Y, Niu L, et al. SGLT2 inhibitors: A novel therapy for cognitive impairment via multifaceted effects on the nervous system. Translational Neurodegeneration. 2024;**13**:41

[43] Cao G, Gong T, Du Y, et al. Mechanism of metformin regulation in central nervous system: Progression and future perspectives. Biomedicine and Pharmacotherapy. 2022;**156**:113686

[44] Yuan Y, Fan X, Guo Z, et al. Metformin protects against spinal cord injury

and cell pyroptosis via AMPK/NLRP3 inflammasome pathway. Analytical Cellular Pathology. 2022;**2022**:1-11

[45] Ruan C, Guo H, Gao J, et al. Neuroprotective effects of metformin on cerebral ischemia-reperfusion injury by regulating PI3K/Akt pathway. Brain and Behavior: A Cognitive Neuroscience Perspective. 2021;**11**(10):e2335. Epub ahead of print 2 October 2021

[46] Kaandorp JJ, van den Broek MPH, Benders MJNL, et al. Rapid target allopurinol concentrations in the hypoxic fetus after maternal administration during labour. Archives of Disease in Childhood. Fetal and Neonatal Edition. 2014;**99**:F144-F148

[47] Gunes T, Ozturk MA, Koklu E, et al. Effect of allopurinol supplementation on nitric oxide levels in asphyxiated newborns. Pediatric Neurology. 2007;**36**:17-24

[48] Engel C, Rüdiger M, Benders MJNL, et al. Detailed statistical analysis plan for ALBINO: Effect of allopurinol in addition to hypothermia for hypoxic-ischemic brain injury on neurocognitive outcome - A blinded randomized placebo-controlled parallel group multicenter trial for superiority (phase III). Trials. 2024;**25**:81

[49] Soliman H, Theret M, Scott W, et al. Multipotent stromal cells: One name, multiple identities. Cell Stem Cell. 2021;**28**:1690-1707

[50] Serrenho I, Rosado M, Dinis A, et al. Stem cell therapy for neonatal hypoxic-ischemic encephalopathy: A systematic review of preclinical studies. International Journal of Molecular Sciences. 2021;**22**:3142

[51] Zhao Y-Q, Xu Y-Y, Zheng Y-M, et al. Human placenta-derived mesenchymal stem cells improve neurological function in rats with intrauterine hypoxic-ischaemic encephalopathy by reducing apoptosis and inflammatory reactions. Frontiers in Bioscience-Landmark. 2024;**29**(4):139. Epub ahead of print 3 April 2024

[52] Teo EJ, Jones LE, Wixey JA, et al. Combined hypothermia and mesenchymal stem cells in animal models of neonatal hypoxic–ischaemic encephalopathy: A systematic review. Pediatric Research. 2022;**92**:25-31

[53] Ranjan AK, Gulati A. Sovateltide mediated endothelin B receptors agonism and curbing neurological disorders. International Journal of Molecular Sciences. 2022;**23**:3146

[54] Gulati A, Adwani SG, Vijaya P, et al. Efficacy and safety of sovateltide in patients with acute cerebral ischaemic stroke: A randomised, double-blind, placebo-controlled, multicentre, phase III clinical trial. Drugs. 2024;**84**:1637-1650

[55] Ramos MD, Briyal S, Prazad P, et al. Neuroprotective effect of sovateltide (IRL 1620, PMZ 1620) in a neonatal rat model of hypoxic-ischemic encephalopathy. Neuroscience. 2022;**480**:194-202

[56] Moustakas D, Mani I, Pouliakis A, et al. The effects of IRL-1620 in post-ischemic brain injury: A systematic review and meta-analysis of experimental studies. Neurocritical Care. 2024;**41**:665-680

[57] Keam SJ. Sovateltide: First approval. Drugs. 2023;**83**:1239-1244

[58] Zhao M, Zhu P, Fujino M, Zhuang J, Guo H, Sheikh I, et al. Oxidative stress in hypoxic-ischemic encephalopathy:

Molecular mechanisms and therapeutic strategies. International Journal of Molecular Sciences. 2016;**17**:2078. DOI: 10.3390/ijms17122078

[59] Kim M, Stepanova A, Niatsetskaya Z, Sosunov S, Arndt S, Murphy MP, et al. Attenuation of oxidative damage by targeting mitochondrial complex I in neonatal hypoxic-ischemic brain injury. Free Radical Biology and Medicine. 2018;**124**:517-524. ISSN 0891-5849

[60] Leaw B, Nair S, Lim R, Thornton C, Mallard C, Hagberg H. Mitochondria, bioenergetics and excitotoxicity: New therapeutic targets in perinatal brain injury. Frontiers in Cellular Neuroscience. 2017;**11**:199. DOI: 10.3389/fncel.2017.00199

Chapter 8

Neonatal General Movements Artificial Intelligence Assessment and Its Clinical Practice

Xinrui Huang, Ming Yi and Tongyan Han

Abstract

General movements assessment (GMA) is an internationally recognized evaluation tool for very early screening and diagnosis of neurological prognosis in high-risk infants. The traditional GMA depends on a few internationally certified doctors, which is also subjective and time-consuming and thus limits its wide use, especially for the newborn. The state-of-the-art methods of intelligent action recognition could automatically extract features of neonatal general movements. Based on the quantitative features, the classification technology with machine learning makes GMA more objective and reliable, making this valuable tool more extensive. This chapter introduces methods of intelligent action recognition and its important applications for GMA, comments on the limitations of these technologies in the past decade, and shares the interdisciplinary views on the future application to improve neonatal health.

Keywords: neonatal development, general movements assessment, artificial intelligence, machine learning, action recognition

1. Introduction

General movements (GMs) are infants' spontaneous movements that offer insights into neurological development [1, 2]. General movements assessment (GMA), as established by Prechtl [3], is vital for early detection of developmental disorders, especially during the writhing phase (0–8 weeks) and fidgety phase (2–5 months), where movement quality can predict future motor outcomes [4], including CP and other motor delays [5, 6]. This method has demonstrated that it is not only crucial in early detection efforts with high reliability and predictive validity [7, 8] but also particularly valuable in low-resource settings, where traditional diagnostic methods may be less accessible [9]. Traditional GMA relies heavily on Gestalt perception, which is also subjective and requires trained assessors to accurately interpret the movements, which can be challenging for less experienced practitioners [4]. Therefore, ongoing training and the development of standardized protocols are essential to ensure the reliability and validity of GMA in clinical practice [10].

Recent advancements in artificial intelligence (AI) have opened new avenues for enhancing the accuracy and efficiency of GMA. AI algorithms can process large datasets of movement patterns, allowing for the identification of subtle abnormalities that may not be easily discernible to the human eye. The integration of AI into GMA not only streamlines the evaluation process but also allows for improving long-term developmental outcomes and enhancing the overall care of neonates by continuously monitoring and analyzing movement patterns [11]. This is particularly beneficial in low-resource settings where access to specialized GMA experts may be limited [9]. These advancements underscore the transformative potential of AI in neonatology, offering opportunities for personalized treatment plans and improved outcomes for vulnerable populations, especially in neonatal intensive care units (NICUs) where early detection and intervention are paramount [12, 13]. The successful implementation of AI-based GMA in clinical practice requires careful consideration of ethical implications, data quality, and interdisciplinary collaboration [14] so that it can ensure that these technologies are developed and validated rigorously to support clinical decision-making effectively and provide immediate feedback to caregivers to enhance the overall quality of care for at-risk infants [4] and simultaneously enhance the applicability of these technologies in clinical settings [8, 12].

To address the challenges and maximize the benefits of the innovative AI-based GMA approaches in neonatal care [8, 15] and ensuring they meet the practical needs of healthcare providers [16], this chapter introduces methods of intelligent action recognition and their important applications for GMA, comments the limitations of these technologies in the past decade and shares the interdisciplinary views on the future application to improve neonatal health.

2. AI-based GMA workflow

The development of standardized protocols for AI-based GMA is essential to ensure consistency and reliability in clinical practice. The SPIRIT-AI extension provides guidelines for clinical trial protocols involving AI interventions, emphasizing the need for clear descriptions of the AI systems used, the data handling processes, and the human-AI interaction dynamics [17]. Generally, the standardized AI-based GMA workflow would involve several key steps: capturing high-quality data of the infant's general movements, preprocessing and annotating the data to enhance clarity, splitting data and applying AI algorithms for training a GMA model, evaluating the model performance and generating reports that summarize the findings for healthcare providers so that the model could be applied in clinical practice. Such a systematic protocol ensures that the AI tools are used effectively and the results are communicated clearly to the clinical team (**Figure 1**).

2.1 Data preparation

2.1.1 Data collection

The nature and availability of the data play a crucial role in GMA. With a growing need for objective GMA in clinical settings and home care, there are currently multiple approaches to capture neonatal GMs, mainly covering sensor-based, vision-based data and the fusion data of different modalities (**Figure 2**).

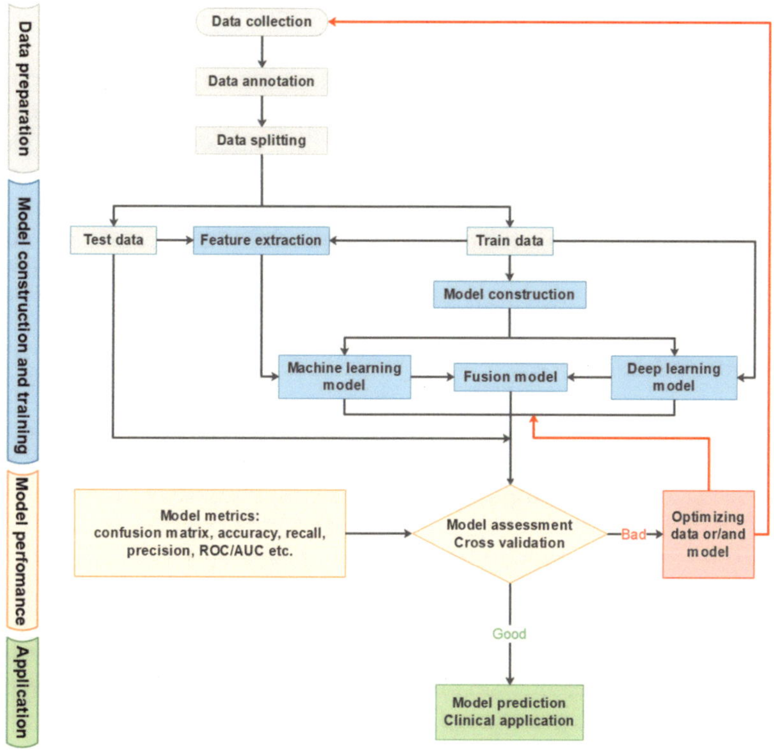

Figure 1.
The overall framework of neonatal general movements artificial intelligence assessment.

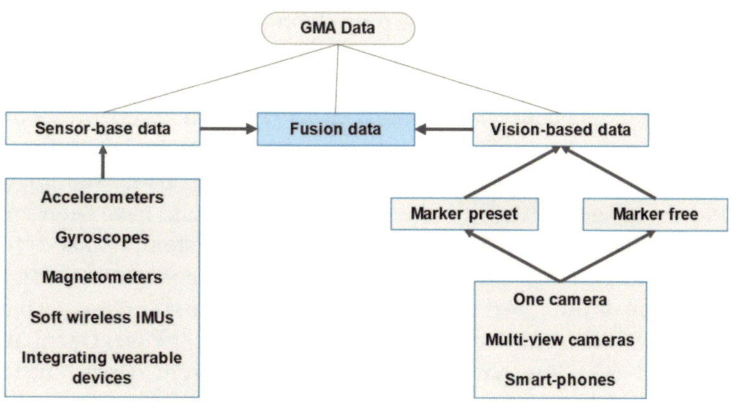

Figure 2.
The GMA data from different collection devices.

2.1.1.1 Sensor-based data

Sensors like accelerometers, gyroscopes, and magnetometers are affordable and small enough so they can be placed on the baby's limbs and record the one-dimensional (1D) signal to track the infant movements [16]. However, these sensors probably disturb the infant movements while the development of ultrathin, soft, and skin-like electronic devices, like soft wireless inertial measurement units (IMUs) [11], can operate wirelessly and adhere gently to the skin, minimizing discomfort for the infant [18], which has paved the way for more comfortable and effective monitoring of neonates in intensive care units and automatically evaluating GMs with quantitative assessments without a clinical observer [9]. Moreover, These wearable sensors extend beyond just monitoring GMs, and they can also facilitate the collection of additional physiological data, such as heart rate variability and metabolic indicators, to gain a holistic view of an infant's health status, which is essential for comprehensive neonatal care [19, 20] and provide complement for GMA [21].

2.1.1.2 Vision-based data

Vision-based data is generally two/three-dimensional (2D/3D) videos or images from different cameras like traditional digital cameras, RGB depth cameras, or smartphones. Traditional RGB cameras have been used over the past few decades for research on human action recognition to capture video sequences. For a study on the infant GMs, a fixed digital camera is generally placed above the infant to record in a supine position where the infant remains awake but not distracted. With advances in imaging technology, RGB depth cameras can simultaneously capture color image sequences and depth maps. Because depth maps are insensitive to changes in illumination conditions, they can provide additional information on body shape and motion and help distinguish projection-like actions from different views [22]. The configuration of multiple cameras can also help distinguish the blocked actions from an individual view by simultaneously capturing the infant GMs from multiple different views [22]. Additionally, the integration of mobile devices into GMA has opened new avenues for remote monitoring and parental involvement [23]. Parents can record their infants' movements at home using smartphones, and the data can then be remotely analyzed by healthcare professionals [24], which not only increases accessibility to GMA but also empowers parents in the developmental monitoring of their children [25, 26].

The vision-based data collection systems either rely on markers preset on certain body parts to record the location of the reflective markers or explore maker-free solutions using image features (e.g., color, shape, and edges) to encode motion information in the videos/images. Although marker-preset techniques have been proven to be relatively accurate in the literature, like the Optitrack system, maker-free methods have become very attractive in the research community of computer vision in the past decade because of not intervening/interfering with the spontaneous movement of the infant [27]. Some open-source toolboxes, such as OpenPose, DeepLabCut, Leap Motion, and MediaPipe, have published several different algorithms for human posture estimation and motion tracking, which can be modified and transferred for infant GMs tracking and anatomic landmark labeling like the ankles, knees, hips, wrists, elbows, shoulders, feet, hands, and face [28].

2.1.1.3 Fusion data

In order to overcome the shortcomings of the above data collection methods and avoid losing data due to environments, occlusion, noise, gestational age, fatigue, etc., the fusion data from a multi-modality system allows consistent evaluation and can enhance the understanding of general movement complexity and variation, which are critical for accurate GMA [4]. For example, for manual annotation purposes, the whole procedure of sensor-based data collection can be recorded by a camera to provide a comprehensive analysis of movement patterns for experts without real-time monitoring. With the development of human pose estimation databases containing various types of movement data sets, the accuracy of pose estimation in video clips can be further improved by using a large amount of training data. This facilitates motion analysis of captured video clips using computer vision methods with portable, low-cost cameras rather than using specific sensors in a traditional way. The neuro-imaging data and other clinical factors like gestational weeks have demonstrated their effectiveness in predicting outcomes [29] and highlighted its utility in neonatal intensive care settings [30, 31]. Therefore, it requires efficient performing and combining work to involve the multi-modality data into GMA decision-making.

2.1.2 Data annotation

To date, AI-based GMA relies heavily on supervised learning, where each data item in the dataset must be assigned an appropriate label, called data annotation. Data annotation describes the process of tagging data to provide the AI algorithm with which part of the data it should identify. A dataset is usually composed of multiple data samples, each containing a set of features and the corresponding target variables after data annotation. For AI-based GMA, generally, each data sample should be annotated by at least three annotators, and to further improve the annotation quality, a majority voting strategy can be used for consistency. Due to its time-consuming and labor-intensive nature, manual data annotation becomes one of the major obstacles in the GMA process. The availability of publicly accessible, tagged datasets will be an important catalyst for driving AI's role in the GMA field. Considering that the data size required for successfully training the GMA AI model are unpredictable and the data annotation process is extremely cumbersome, the introduction of semi-supervised and unsupervised learning algorithms for annotation in future studies could at least slightly facilitate, accelerate, and reduce the cost of the data preparation process.

2.1.3 Data splitting

Data splitting is an indispensable step in the development of AI models. Before splitting the data set, the data needs to be cleaned to eliminate the effects of outliers, missing values, and duplicate values on the model. The quality and proportion of dataset partitioning directly affect the training effect and prediction performance of the model. Therefore, the proportion and method of data splitting need to be carefully selected to ensure the practicality and generalization ability of the model. Common methods for splitting data are as follows: (1) Random splitting: the data set is randomly divided into training set, validation set, and test set, which is suitable for large datasets and uniform feature distribution. (2) Stratified sampling splitting: according to the distribution of target variables, the dataset is divided into different layers, and then samples are extracted from each layer to form the training set, validation set, and test set, which can ensure similar data distribution between the sets. (3) Set aside splitting: first, divide the dataset into the training set and the test set, and then use the training set to further divide the validation set, which can be used for both model selection and parameter adjustment.

The choice of dataset partition proportions usually depends on the size of the data and the complexity of the model. In general, the proportion of the training set should be larger than the proportion of the test set to ensure that the model has enough data for training and learning. Common divisions include 70% training set, 30% test set, 80% training set, and 20% test set. The training set is the dataset used during the model training process, which contains all the features and label information needed for the model learning. Through the training set, the model can learn the distribution and rules of the data so as to adjust its own parameters to achieve the optimal prediction effect. The test set is the data set that is used to evaluate the model performance, which does not participate in the training process of the model and is only used to verify the predictive ability of the model on unknown data. Through the test set, the generalization ability of the model can be evaluated to determine whether the model can make accurate predictions on the new data.

2.2 Model construction and training

Constructing and training the proper GMA AI model involves many aspects such as choosing the appropriate model structure and tuning and optimizing model parameters. However, the construction and training of AI models are not done once and for all and require continuous improvement and tuning. Therefore, it is crucial for researchers and clinical practitioners to continuously learn and master these techniques and methods.

2.2.1 Model construction

As mentioned above, most of the existing literature treats GMA as a supervised rather than an unsupervised classification. The models are generally divided into three categories according to the network functions: traditional machine learning models, deep learning models, and fusion models. The comparison of these three models is presented in **Table 1**. More details are introduced as follows.

2.2.1.1 Machine learning models

Traditional machine learning models use hand-crafted feature extraction techniques combined with classifiers, which have been used for action recognition for quite a long time and with considerable success. To identify important features to achieve powerful medical functions, it is necessary to work closely together for data scientists and clinicians to acquire considerable domain expertise. For sensor-based data or marker trajectories tracked from vision-based data, features like movement centroid, velocity, frequency, acceleration and variability have demonstrated good predictors of CP in machine learning models [32]. The high-level features of structured information relevant to the actions in vision-based data like optical flow and directional gradient histogram (HOG) have also achieved good permanence for CP in addition to the low-level features like corners, edges, or contours in the images. The classifiers are used to make decisions or diagnosis based on input features; the choice of the classifiers depends on many factors, such as feature type, feature size, and the computation resources available. Currently, the classifiers used in traditional machine learning models are mainly native Bayes (NB), linear discriminant analysis (LDA), quadratic discriminant analysis (QDA), logistic regression (LR), support vector machine (SVM), K-nearest neighbor (KNN), decision tree (DT), random forest (RF), AdaBoost, LogitBoost, XGBoost, Log-linearization Gaussian mixed network (LLGMN), and partial least squares regression (PLSR).

Models	Advantages	Disadvantages
Machine learning models	The features used to train the model are clearly known. Less data is required for training. Calculation time and memory usage are low. The models are easily understood.	Effective and accurate feature detectors and extraction methods are usually required. Due to the high feature dimension, the feature selection and dimension reduction method may be required. Data preprocessing and standardization are often required for significant performance. Recognition ability is generally low, and management of inter-and intra-class problems is inefficient.
Deep learning models	No professional knowledge is needed to extract the features; Features are not manually designed and can be learned directly from the raw data; Deep neural network can extract deep high-level features, which is more suitable for complex tasks. Hierarchical and translation-invariant features can be obtained from the model to solve the inter-class and intra-class problems. It is not mandatory to require data preprocessing and normalization to achieve high performance.	Needs to collect massive data will result in lacking suitable datasets. Model training requires a large amount of data to avoid overfitting. Model training is time-consuming and requires advanced, powerful computing resources to accelerate the training process. The generalization ability of the model should be considered.
Fusion models	Features can be expressed from different aspects. The dataset consists of data from multi-modality devices. The results generated by using multi-source information fusion are more accurate.	Model construction will be more complex and challenging. Large datasets need to be processed, and the training time may be longer. Demand for computing resources will increase significantly.

Table 1.
Comparison of three types of AI models.

2.2.1.2 Deep learning models

The hand-crafted feature extraction methods are complex to build and difficult to modify, which hampers the ability of the traditional machine learning model to provide a unified global solution to new datasets. Deep learning models can automatically learn the features and classify them by using deep networks to complete the feature extraction and classification tasks. Thus, the deep learning models save time and effort and can also prevent the loss of potentially useful features that might be ignored by hand-crafted feature extraction. The most famous supervised techniques for GMA include convolutional neural network (CNN), long and short-term memory (LSTM). These deep learning methods are designed to learn complex problems in an end-to-end manner. For example, for vision-based data, the raw videos/images can be directly input into the CNN and the CNN uses a feature detector called a kernel or filter to scan the images to check for the presence of a specific feature, a process called convolution, which thus capture the spatial and temporal dependence in the image to better enable the model to understand the complexity of the image. The LSTM contains a storage mechanism or "memory" for saving information from a previous input, which affects the output of subsequent layers. Given that the GMA video is essentially a form of sequential data, LSTM uses temporal information in the video to effectively capture sequential dynamics for accurate GMs identification.

2.2.1.3 Fusion models

To improve the accuracy and stability of the GMA classification model, a fusion model can be constructed to ensure the better overall performance of the data. The GMA fusion model can be built by decision fusion and feature fusion. The decision fusion method is designed to mix the multiple results of various classification algorithms/models into a result called an integrated decision to make a single final decision. Among them, majority voting is a general way to integrate different ways of results. For different classification models, the category with the most votes is the final result. Other commonly used model fusion methods are the weighted average method, Bagging, etc. The feature fusion method is to combine various model features into the high-dimensional feature vectors to train and test the classifier. The literature shows that feature fusion methods have higher performance compared to decision fusion methods. The feature fusion method can raise problems such as dimension disasters and missing data due to device unavailability at a given time, which need to be managed by using dimensionality reduction and interpolation techniques, such as principal component analysis (PCA) and autoencoder.

2.2.2 Model training

Model training is to constantly adjust the model parameters and minimize the prediction error to make the model reach the equilibrium point of model fitting ability and generalization ability. Fitting ability refers to the performance of model on known data (training set); generalization ability refers to the performance of model on unknown data (test set). Common model training skills: (1) Adjust hyperparameters: The methods for hyperparameter adjustment include grid search, random search, and Bayesian optimization. By adjusting the hyperparameters, such as learning rate, number of iterations, the optimal model configuration can be found. (2) Early stopping method: During the model training process, if the loss or accuracy of the validation set no longer improves, the training will be stopped, which can effectively prevent overfitting and improve the generalization ability of the model. (3) Integrated learning: Integrated learning is a method to improve the overall performance by combining the prediction results of multiple models. Common integrated learning algorithms include random forest, gradient lifting tree, etc. (4) Regularization: Regularization is to constrain the complexity of a model by adding penalty terms to reduce the risk of overfitting. Common regularization methods include L1 regularization and L2 regularization.

2.3 Model performance assessment

After model training, we finally got a so-called "optimal solution," but how to prove that this optimal solution is the true optimal solution? We need to assess the model performance to confirm the truth of this "optimal solution." Model performance is generally evaluated by the performance indicators and stability indicators of the model. Generally, accuracy, precision, recall and F1 score, AUC and other evaluation indicators are used to judge the performance of the classification model (**Figure 3**). Model stability refers to how long the model performance can last, and the PSI index is generally used to evaluate the stability of the model. Cross-validation (CV) is a method to evaluate the model performance by splitting the data sets into multiple subsets and training and verifying the models multiple times on these subsets, such as K-fold cross-validation, where the data are randomly divided into k equal-size sets; this training-validation cycle was repeated k times, each alternating with the validation set; the final overall performance is the average of k times of performance (**Figure 4**). The overall performance of the classification model can commonly be presented with the confusion matrix, which forms the basis of precision (positive predictive value), recall (sensitivity), and accuracy. When K equals the number of training sets, K-fold cross-validation becomes leave-one-out cross-validation (LOO-CV), which is commonly used in small-size training sets.

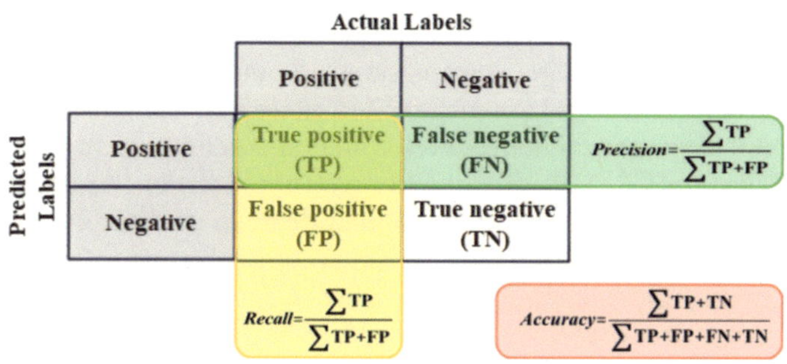

Figure 3.
Common metrics to evaluate the classification model performance.

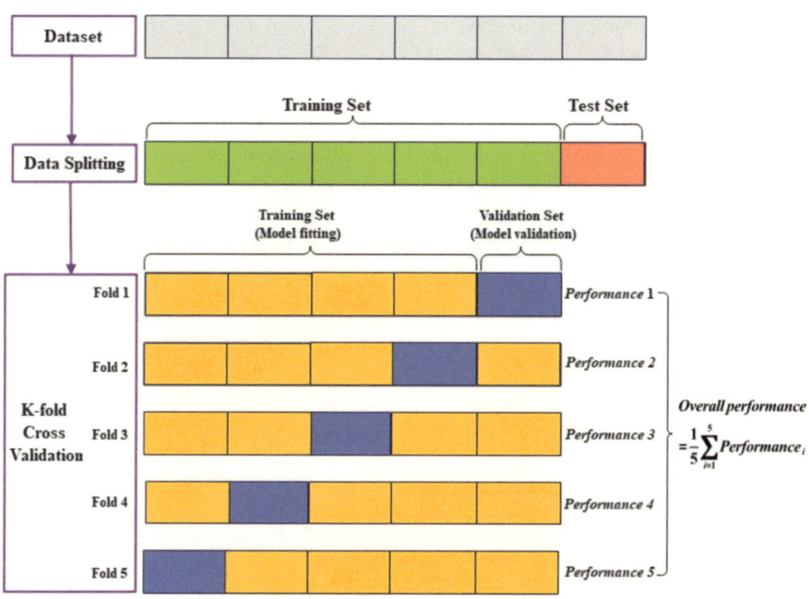

Figure 4.
K-fold cross-validation (K = 5).

3. AI-based GMA for clinical practice

3.1 Clinical application

In clinical practice, GMA is utilized to monitor the GMs of infants from early fetal life until the end of the first half-year after birth [2, 6]. The GMA's ability to predict long-term neurodevelopmental outcomes is further supported by findings that abnormal GMs are linked with clinical features such as preterm birth and low birth weight [33]. Infants with congenital heart disease (CHD) exhibited a higher percentage of normal suboptimal movements [34], while those with fetal operated myelomeningocele (MMC) [35] and suffering Perinatal stroke (PS) [36] showed a significant risk for abnormal GMs. The predictive value of the GM assessment is particularly significant in populations undergoing neonatal surgery, where the risk of developmental disabilities is heightened [1]. GMA is a valuable tool for the early detection of atypical development that is critical for the diagnosis of congenital motor disorders and neurodevelopmental disorders to ensure timely access to early intervention services to improve motor outcomes (e.g., coordination and posture) and support other areas of development (e.g., social and language) [7, 9]. Research has shown that the GMA is effective in predicting atypical neurodevelopmental outcomes in various populations of infants [37], such as CP [1, 9, 38], autism spectrum disorder (ASD), Rett syndrome (RTT) [6, 35], and also effective in evaluation of diseases or clinical conditions including seizure activity [39] and resuscitation monitorization [40].

According to the infant's age, GMs vary in order, speed, and amplitude in three important phases, that is preterm phase (28–36/38 gestational weeks) or writhing phase (36/38–46/52 gestational weeks) and fidgety movement phase (46/50–55/60 gestational weeks) [9]. Thus, three sub-types of abnormal GMs in preterm or writhing phase can be distinguished as monotonous GMs (monotonous movement order and movement speed and amplitude changes reduced), cramped-synchronized GMs (whole-body muscle contraction and relaxation with periods of synchronous) and chaotic GMs (extreme lack of movement fluency as well as large amplitude of movements). Fidgety movements (FMs) should be smaller in amplitude, and higher in speed, than writhing movements. Thus, there are two sub-types of abnormal GMs in the fidgety movement phase, which are absent and present FMs with very large amplitude and excessively fast and jerky speeds [41]. The above features of GMs underscore the potential for AI to assist GMA in identifying these abnormalities through pattern recognition and predictive analytics [12], which presents a promising avenue for enhancing neonatal care [42, 43]. **Table 2** shows the different AI models for using various GMA data to predict atypical development, which exhibited sensitivity and specificity comparable to clinical traditional measures like neuroimaging [1, 2].

3.2 Clinical limitation and solutions

Although AI-based GMA has shown excellent results, there are still many limitations and challenges that hinder its widespread use in clinical settings. One significant limitation is the variability in the interpretation of GMs among clinicians. GMA data annotation relies heavily on the subjective judgment of trained professionals, which can lead to inconsistencies in diagnostic accuracy and predictive validity across different settings [7]. For instance, the criteria for what constitutes "normal" or "abnormal" GMs can differ significantly between different clinicians and studies, making it challenging to establish a normative reference standard [59]. Another limitation is that the data size used in current AI-based GMA models is relatively small, and the data collected generally focuses on specific gestational age groups, which may not adequately represent the full spectrum of neonatal development. This lack of comprehensive data can hinder the ability of the AI-based GMA models to generalize findings

AI models	Clinical application	Main ideas	Data information	Model performance
Machine learning models	PS infants screening [36]	Feature: optical flow Classifier: SVM	Accelerometer data: 21 typical infants and 13 PS infants	Accuracy 75%
	Spastic CP [44]	Feature: inter-body part angles, age, stride length, and leg length Classifier: NB, LR, DT, LDA, kNN, SVM	IMU sensor data: 15 healthy infants and 28 spastic CP infants	Accuracy using SVM 88%
	Neuromotor disease [28]	Feature: time and frequency features from body keypoint trajectory Classifier: DT, NB, SVM, kNN, RF, LR, gradient boosting, and voting classifier	RGB videos: 37 normal GMs and 66 abnormal GMs from 96 neonates	Accuracy 93.33%; precision 93.75; recall 93.75; F1–93.33%, and AUC-ROC 1.000
	CP [45]	Feature: optical flow Classifier: SVM	RGB videos: 15 infants with CP, 67 infants without CP	10-fold CV, Accuracy 93%
	CP [46]	Feature: Large displacement optical flow + infant body shape Classifier: LR, AdaBoost, LogitBoost, RF	RGB videos: 98 typical infants, 29 atypical infants	LOO-CV, GMA Accuracy using AdaBoost 85.83%; CP Accuracy using RF 92.13%
	CP [47]	Feature: histogram of posture Classifier: KNN, LDA, ensemble	MINI-RGBD public dataset	LOO-CV, Accuracy using ensemble 91.67%
	CP [48]	Feature: angle, velocity, symmetry Classifier: SVM, DT, XGBoost, extra-tree, neural network	MINI-RGBD and RVI-38 datasets	Accuracy for MINI-RGBD 92%; Accuracy for RVI-38 97.37%
	CP [49]	Feature: infant body shape Classifier: LLGMN	4-class videos from 21infants	Accuracy for normal/abnormal 90.2%; Accuracy for four classes 83.1%
	Neuromotor disease [50]	Feature: joint trajectory Classifier: NB	RGB videos: 19 high-risk infants, 85 healthy infants	Significant difference in NB scores
Deep learning models	Neuromotor disease [51]	Self-supervised spatiotemporal attention network	Multi-view RGB videos: 62 normal writhing movements, 108 abnormal monotonic movements	Accuracy 87.06 ± 4.51; Sensitivity 89.55 ± 8.34; Specificity 84.45 ± 15.19
	CP [52]	Keras VGG19 transfer-learning model + LSTM	RGB videos: 135 healthy infants, 80 infants with CP	10-fold CV, Accuracy 65.1%

AI models	Clinical application	Main ideas	Data information	Model performance
Fusion models	CP [53]	Feature: optical flow and trajectory features from videos + data features from motion sensors Classifier: SVM	RGB videos: 14 infants with CP, 64 infants without CP	Accuracy 87%
	CP [54]	Feature: frequency features from videos and sensors Classifier: PLSR	RGB videos: 14 infants with CP, 64 infants without CP	CV, Accuracy 91%
	CP [55]	Feature: body keypoint trajectory + discrete wavelet transform features Classifier: stacking with SVM, RF, AdaBoost, XGBoost	RGB videos: 60 normal infants, 60 abnormal infants	Accuracy 93.3%
	CP [56]	Joint trajectory + spatiotemporal attention model	RGB videos: 235 infants with/without FMs	ROC-AUC 81.87%
	ASD [57]	Skeleton keypoint trajectory + CNN-LSTM network	RGB videos: 169 infants with ASD, 68 typical infants	Accuracy 80.9%
	ASD [58]	Feature: Shoulder and head posture features + response duration Classifier: PyTorch deep learning frame	RGB videos: 29 infants with ASD, 1 typical infant	Accuracy 93.3%
	Seizure monitoring [39]	Feature: movement of the anatomic landmarks Classifier: LR, SVM, XGBoost	Videos linked to electroencephalograms (video-EEG data) from 115 infants	5-fold CV, ROC-AUCs of XGBoost for sedation (0.90, 0.91, 0.87); for cerebral dysfunction (0.91, 0.90, 0.76)

Table 2.
Clinical application of the AI-based GMA.

and apply them in broader clinical practices [60]. Moreover, for real-time manipulation, current AI models still require powerful and expensive computation resources like GPU and TPU, which limits their usability in clinical. Finally, the integration of advanced technologies and statistical methods into the GMA process is still in its infancy [11], which needs time to enhance the clinicians' comprehensive understanding and embrace these innovations to ensure better outcomes for at-risk infants.

To easily integrate AI-based GMA into routine clinical practice and provide pediatricians and therapists with a straightforward method to monitor infant development, several efforts could be involved: (1) for data collection, multi-modality datasets should be collected, but the data collection system is as simple as possible [61]. Simple system could minimize the preparation work on infants with minimum clinical workers. Moreover, the data collection system should be easily setup in a comfortable environment to ensure the safety of the infants and simultaneously reduce the infants GMA data loss because of interference sources, background clutter, viewpoint changes, and occlusion [62]. (2) for data annotation, standardized training and certification for clinicians performing GMA is necessary to consist of the GMA results. (3) For the AI-based models, extracting features and processing of data, especially for video files, is still complex and time consuming, making it less accessible for clinicians as a rapid clinical measurement tool. Further research is needed to design and develop a platform or software in a more user-friendly and accurate manner, thus further expanding its clinical application and meeting specific clinical needs. Additionally, transfer learning could be used to train the AI-based models with new datasets from the pre-trained models rather than train from scratch, which can help reduce the training time and improve the model performance.

4. Future prospect

As research continues to evolve, the prospects of AI-based GMA are promising. One significant area for future exploration is the application of GMA in diverse populations, including those in low- and middle-income countries. The assessment's high sensitivity and specificity make it an ideal candidate for implementation in resource-limited settings, where early identification of neurodevelopmental issues can lead to timely interventions [9]. Expanding studies on GMA in these regions could provide valuable insights and improve outcomes for vulnerable populations [9].

Another promising avenue is the use of technology to streamline the GMA process and provide a more comprehensive understanding of an infant's developmental trajectory [1], which could facilitate better prognostication and individualized care plans for infants undergoing surgical procedures or those diagnosed with neonatal encephalopathy [1, 7]. Advances in video analysis and machine learning could automate the assessment, making GMA more accessible and reducing the variability associated with human assessors. This technological integration could also enable remote assessments, further broadening the reach of GMA in clinical practice. Given the achievements of deep learning and their accuracy in detecting people and objects, with the development of data enhancement and different transfer-learning methods, the number of video/image databases of different GM types is expected to increase, and large public datasets annotated by experts will be an important catalyst for driving AI role in GMA. Additionally, to adequately train AI models, large and diverse datasets are needed and thus legal issues and regulations surrounding patient data access will arise, which makes consider to develop privacy protection technology to hide the identity of the patients.

Finally, ongoing research should also focus on understanding the underlying mechanisms that contribute to abnormal GMs. Identifying specific biomarkers or neurophysiological correlates could enhance the predictive power of GMA and inform targeted interventions [63]. As we continue to refine our understanding of early motor/neural development, the AI-based GMA will likely play a pivotal role in shaping future practices in neonatal care.

5. Conclusions

GMA plays a vital role in early detection and intervention strategies for infants at risk of developmental challenges. The ongoing research and application of the AI-based GMA underscore its importance in pediatric healthcare and developmental neuroscience since it can offer numerous advantages, including its non-invasive nature and high predictive validity for neurodevelopmental disorders. As AI systems become more integrated into clinical workflows, the collaboration between human intelligence and AI will be vital in making informed decisions regarding patient care. This chapter introduces methods of intelligent action recognition and its important applications for GMA, comments on the limitations of current technologies in the past decade, and shares interdisciplinary views on the future application to improve neonatal health.

Acknowledgements

This work is supported by the Beijing Natural Science Foundation (4242004, L222016), the Peking University Health Science Center Medical Education Research Funding Project (2022YB17), the Open Research Fund of the National Center for Protein Sciences at Peking University in Beijing (KF-202402), and the National Natural Science Foundation of China (32271053).

Author details

Xinrui Huang[1,2]*, Ming Yi[2,3] and Tongyan Han[4]

1 Department of Biophysics, School of Basic Medical Sciences, Peking University, Beijing, China

2 Key Laboratory for Neuroscience, Ministry of Education/National Health Commission, Beijing, China

3 Neuroscience Reasearch Institute, Peking University, Beijing, China

4 Department of Pediatrics, Third Hospital, Peking University, Beijing, China

*Address all correspondence to: huangxr@pku.edu.cn

References

[1] Crowle C, Galea C, Walker K, Novak I, Badawi N. Prediction of neurodevelopment at one year of age using the general movements assessment in the neonatal surgical population. Early Human Development. 2018;**118**:42-47. DOI: 10.1016/j.earlhumdev.2018.02.001

[2] Crowle C, Loughran Fowlds A, Novak I, Badawi N. Use of the general movements assessment for the early detection of cerebral palsy in infants with congenital anomalies requiring surgery. Journal of Clinical Medicine. 2019;**8**(9):1286. DOI: 10.3390/jcm8091286

[3] Einspieler C, Prechtl HF. Prechtl's assessment of general movements: A diagnostic tool for the functional assessment of the young nervous system. Mental Retardation and Developmental Disabilities Research Reviews. 2005;**11**(1):61-67. DOI: 10.1002/mrdd.20051

[4] Wu YC, van Rijssen IM, Buurman MT, Dijkstra LJ, Hamer EG, Hadders-Algra M. Temporal and spatial localisation of general movement complexity and variation-why gestalt assessment requires experience. Acta Paediatrica. 2021;**110**(1):290-300. DOI: 10.1111/apa.15300

[5] Gima H, Nakamura T. Association between general movements assessment and later motor delay (excluding cerebral palsy) in low-birth-weight infants. Brain Sciences. 2022;**12**(6):686. DOI: 10.3390/brainsci12060686

[6] Einspieler C, Sigafoos J, Bölte S, Bratl-Pokorny KD, Landa R, Marschik PB. Highlighting the first 5 months of life: General movements in infants later diagnosed with autism spectrum disorder or Rett syndrome. Research in Autism Spectrum Disorder. 2014;**8**(3):286-291. DOI: 10.1016/j.rasd.2013.12.013

[7] Seesahai J, Luther M, Rhoden CC, Church PT, Asztalos E, Banihani R. The general movements assessment in term and late-preterm infants diagnosed with neonatal encephalopathy, as a predictive tool of cerebral palsy by 2 years of age: A scoping review protocol. Systematic Reviews. 2020;**9**(1):154. DOI: 10.1186/s13643-020-01358-x

[8] Seesahai J, Luther M, Church PT, Maddalena P, Asztalos E, Rotter T, et al. The assessment of general movements in term and late-preterm infants diagnosed with neonatal encephalopathy, as a predictive tool of cerebral palsy by 2 years of age-a scoping review. Systematic Reviews. 2021;**10**(1):226. DOI: 10.1186/s13643-021-01765-8

[9] Tomantschger I, Herrero D, Einspieler C, Hamamura C, Voos MC, Marschik PB. The general movement assessment in non-European low- and middle-income countries. Revista de Saúde Pública. 2018;**52**:6. DOI: 10.11606/s1518-8787.2018052000332

[10] Leyener U, Kraushaar C, Dathe AK, Felderhoff-Müser U, Marschik PB, Zhang D, et al. Physiotherapy in German neonatal intensive care units - indication and clinical application of the general movements assessments. Zeitschrift für Geburtshilfe und Neonatologie. 2022;**226**(4):256-264. DOI: 10.1055/a-1791-5778

[11] Bao B, Zhang S, Li H, Cui W, Guo K, Zhang Y, et al. Intelligence sparse sensor network for automatic early evaluation of general movements in infants. Advanced Science.

2024;**11**(19):e2306025. DOI: 10.1002/advs.202306025

[12] Sullivan BA, Kausch SL, Fairchild KD. Artificial and human intelligence for early identification of neonatal sepsis. Pediatric Research. 2023;**93**(2):350-356. DOI: 10.1038/s41390-022-02274-7

[13] Micali G, Corallo F, Pagano M, Giambò FM, Duca A, D'Aleo P, et al. Artificial intelligence and heart-brain connections: A narrative review on algorithms utilization in clinical practice. Healthcare. 2024;**12**(14):1380. Available from: https://www.mdpi.com/2227-9032/12/14/1380

[14] Sullivan BA, Beam K, Vesoulis ZA, Aziz KB, Husain AN, Knake LA, et al. Transforming neonatal care with artificial intelligence: Challenges, ethical consideration, and opportunities. Journal of Perinatology. 2024;**44**(1):1-11. DOI: 10.1038/s41372-023-01848-5

[15] Ferronato PAM, Resende B, Manoel EJ. Interweaving social and manipulative development in early infancy: Some direction for infant caregiving. Infant Behavior & Development. 2021;**63**:101564. DOI: 10.1016/j.infbeh.2021.101564

[16] Clark CCT, Bisi MC, Duncan MJ, Stagni R. Technology-based methods for the assessment of fine and gross motor skill in children: A systematic overview of available solutions and future steps for effective in-field use. Journal of Sports Sciences. 2021;**39**(11):1236-1276. DOI: 10.1080/02640414.2020.1864984

[17] Cruz Rivera S, Liu X, Chan A-W, Denniston AK, Calvert MJ, Darzi A, et al. Guidelines for clinical trial protocols for interventions involving artificial intelligence: The SPIRIT-AI extension. Nature Medicine. 2020;**26**(9):1351-1363. DOI: 10.1038/s41591-020-1037-7

[18] Chung HU, Kim BH, Lee JY, Lee J, Xie Z, Ibler EM, et al. Binodal, wireless epidermal electronic systems with in-sensor analytics for neonatal intensive care. Science. 2019;**363**(6430):eaau0780. DOI: 10.1126/science.aau0780

[19] Palmer AR, Distefano R, Leneman K, Berry D. Reliability of the BodyGuard2 (FirstBeat) in the detection of heart rate variability. Applied Psychophysiology and Biofeedback. 2021;**46**(3):251-258. DOI: 10.1007/s10484-021-09510-6

[20] Gao W, Brooks GA, Klonoff DC. Wearable physiological systems and technologies for metabolic monitoring. Journal of Applied Physiology. 1985;**124**(3):548-556. DOI: 10.1152/japplphysiol.00407.2017

[21] Sitaula C, Grooby E, Kwok TC, Sharkey D, Marzbanrad F, Malhotra A. Artificial intelligence-driven wearable technologies for neonatal cardiorespiratory monitoring. Part 2: Artificial intelligence. Pediatric Research. 2023;**93**(2):426-436. DOI: 10.1038/s41390-022-02417-w

[22] Clark RA, Mentiplay BF, Hough E, Pua YH. Three-dimensional cameras and skeleton pose tracking for physical function assessment: A review of uses, validity, current developments and Kinect alternatives. Gait & Posture. 2019;**68**:193-200. DOI: 10.1016/j.gaitpost.2018.11.029

[23] Balta D, Kuo H, Wang J, Porco IG, Morozova O, Schladen MM, et al. Characterization of Infants' general movements using a commercial RGB-depth sensor and a deep neural network tracking processing tool: An exploratory study. Sensors (Basel). 2022;**22**(19):7426. DOI: 10.3390/s22197426

[24] Kukka AJ, Sundelin HEK, Basnet O, Paudel P, Upadhyay

Subedi K, Svensson K, et al. NeuroMotion smartphone application for remote general movements assessment: A feasibility study in Nepal. BMJ Open. 2024;**14**(3):e080063. DOI: 10.1136/bmjopen-2023-080063

[25] Boonzaaijer M, van Wesel F, Nuysink J, Volman MJM, Jongmans MJ. A home-video method to assess infant gross motor development: Parent perspectives on feasibility. BMC Pediatrics. 2019;**19**(1):392. DOI: 10.1186/s12887-019-1779-x

[26] Sardi L, Idri A, Redman LM, Alami H, Bezad R, Fernández-Alemán JL. Mobile health applications for postnatal care: Review and analysis of functionalities and technical features. Computer Methods and Programs in Biomedicine. 2020;**184**:105114. DOI: 10.1016/j.cmpb.2019.105114

[27] D'Haene M, Chorin F, Colson SS, Guérin O, Zory R, Piche E. Validation of a 3D Markerless motion capture tool using multiple pose and depth estimations for quantitative gait analysis. Sensors. 2024;**24**(22):7105. Available from: https://www.mdpi.com/1424-8220/24/22/7105

[28] Huang X, Huang C, Yin W, Huang H, Xie Z, Huang Y, et al. Automatic quantitative intelligent assessment of neonatal general movements with video tracking. Displays. 2024;**82**:102658. DOI: 10.1016/j.displa.2024.102658

[29] de Mendonça KT, de Souza Pascoal AF, Lanza FC, Viñolas Prat B, de Souza Morais RL, Resende Camargos AC. Clinical factors related to abnormal general movements trajectories: Development of a multicriteria index. Pediatric Physical Therapy. 2024;**36**(4):440-447. DOI: 10.1097/pep.0000000000001129

[30] Li A, Mullin S, Elkin PL. Improving prediction of survival for extremely premature infants born at 23 to 29 weeks gestational age in the neonatal intensive care unit: Development and evaluation of machine learning models. JMIR Medical Informatics. 2024;**12**:e42271. DOI: 10.2196/42271

[31] Van Laere D, Meeus M, Beirnaert C, Sonck V, Laukens K, Mahieu L, et al. Machine learning to support hemodynamic intervention in the neonatal intensive care unit. Clinics in Perinatology. 2020;**47**(3):435-448. DOI: 10.1016/j.clp.2020.05.002

[32] Cahill-Rowley K, Schadl K, Vassar R, Yeom KW, Stevenson DK, Rose J. Prediction of gait impairment in toddlers born preterm from near-term brain microstructure assessed with DTI, using exhaustive feature selection and cross-validation. Frontiers in Human Neuroscience. 2019;**13**:305. DOI: 10.3389/fnhum.2019.00305

[33] Mallmann GS, França ALN, Almeida PR, Oliveira LS, Merey LSF, Soares-Marangoni DA. Association between the general movement optimality score and clinical features in newborns during hospitalization: A cross-sectional study. Early Human Development. 2023;**177-178**:105720. DOI: 10.1016/j.earlhumdev.2023.105720

[34] Huisenga DC, la Bastide-van GS, Van Bergen AH, Sweeney JK, Hadders-Algra M. Predictive value of general movements assessment for developmental delay at 18 months in children with complex congenital heart disease. Early Human Development. 2024;**188**:105916. DOI: 10.1016/j.earlhumdev.2023.105916

[35] Cott R, Hagmann C, Etter R, Latal B. Differences in the distribution of the general movements

classification between neonatal risk groups in the Children's hospital Zurich: An observational study. Zeitschrift für Geburtshilfe und Neonatologie. 2022;**226**(4):265-273. DOI: 10.1055/a-1808-2843

[36] Gao Y, Long Y, Guan Y, Basu A, Baggaley J, Ploetz T. Towards reliable, automated general movement assessment for perinatal stroke screening in infants using wearable accelerometers. The Proceedings of the ACM on Interactive, Mobile, Wearable and Ubiquitous Technologies. 2019;**3**(1):12. DOI: 10.1145/3314399

[37] Hadders-Algra M, Tacke U, Pietz J, Rupp A, Philippi H. Predictive value of the general movements assessment and standardized infant NeuroDevelopmental assessment in infants at high risk of neurodevelopmental disorders. Developmental Medicine and Child Neurology. 2024;**66**(10):1361-1368. DOI: 10.1111/dmcn.15901

[38] Peinado-Gorlat P, Gómez de Valcárcel-Sabater M, Gorlat-Sánchez B. General movement assessment as a tool for determining the prognosis in infantile cerebral palsy in preterm infants: A systematic review. Revista de Neurologia. 2020;**71**(4):134-142. DOI: 10.33588/rn.7104.2019460

[39] Gleason A, Richter F, Beller N, Arivazhagan N, Feng R, Holmes E, et al. Detection of neurologic changes in critically ill infants using deep learning on video data: A retrospective single center cohort study. EClinicalMedicine. 2024;**78**:102919. DOI: 10.1016/j.eclinm.2024.102919

[40] Fortunov RM, Cabacungan E, Barry JS, Jagarapu J. Artificial intelligence and informatics in neonatal resuscitation. Seminars in Perinatology. 2024;**48**(8):151992. DOI: 10.1016/j.semperi.2024.151992

[41] Sokołów M, Adde L, Klimont L, Pilarska E, Einspieler C. Early intervention and its short-term effect on the temporal organization of fidgety movements. Early Human Development. 2020;**151**:105197. DOI: 10.1016/j.earlhumdev.2020.105197

[42] Diakiw SM, Hall JMM, VerMilyea M, Lim AYX, Quangkananurug W, Chanchamroen S, et al. An artificial intelligence model correlated with morphological and genetic features of blastocyst quality improves ranking of viable embryos. Reproductive Biomedicine Online. 2022;**45**(6):1105-1117. DOI: 10.1016/j.rbmo.2022.07.018

[43] Yuge M, Marschik PB, Nakajima Y, Yamori Y, Kanda T, Hirota H, et al. Movements and postures of infants aged 3 to 5 months: To what extent is their optimality related to perinatal events and to the neurological outcome? Early Human Development. 2011;**87**(3):231-237. DOI: 10.1016/j.earlhumdev.2010.12.046

[44] Sukhadia N, Kamboj P. IMU-based approach to detect spastic cerebral palsy in infants at early stages. EAI Endorsed Transactions on Pervasive Health and Technology. 2024;**10**:1-12. DOI: 10.4108/eetpht.10.5258

[45] Stahl A, Schellewald C, Stavdahl Ø, Aamo OM, Adde L, Kirkerød H. An optical flow-based method to predict infantile cerebral palsy. IEEE Transactions on Neural Systems and Rehabilitation Engineering. 2012;**20**(4):605-614. DOI: 10.1109/tnsre.2012.2195030

[46] Orlandi S, Raghuram K, Smith CR, Mansueto D, Church P, Shah V, et al. Detection of atypical and typical infant

movements using computer-based video analysis. Annual International Conference of the IEEE Engineering in Medicine and Biology Society. 2018;**2018**:3598-3601. DOI: 10.1109/embc.2018.8513078

[47] McCay KD, Ho ESL, Marcroft C, Embleton ND. Establishing pose based features using histograms for the detection of abnormal infant movements. In: 41st Annual International Conference of the IEEE Engineering in Medicine and Biology Society (EMBC). Vol. 2019. 2019. pp. 5469-5472. DOI: 10.1109/embc.2019.8857680

[48] Ali MM, Mohamed SI. A pose estimation for motion tracking of infants cerebral palsy. Multimedia Tools and Applications. 2024;**4**:1-26. DOI: 10.1007/s11042-024-19198-5

[49] Tsuji T, Nakashima S, Hayashi H, Soh Z, Furui A, Shibanoki T, et al. Markerless measurement and evaluation of general movements in infants. Scientific Reports. 2020;**10**(1):1422. DOI: 10.1038/s41598-020-57580-z

[50] Chambers C, Seethapathi N, Saluja R, Loeb H, Pierce SR, Bogen DK, et al. Computer vision to automatically assess infant Neuromotor risk. IEEE Transactions on Neural Systems and Rehabilitation Engineering. 2020;**28**(11):2431-2442. DOI: 10.1109/TNSRE.2020.3029121

[51] Yin W, Chen L, Huang X, Huang C, Wang Z, Bian Y, et al. A self-supervised spatio-temporal attention network for video-based 3D infant pose estimation. Medical Image Analysis. 2024;**96**:103208. DOI: 10.1016/j.media.2024.103208

[52] Schmidt W, Regan M, Fahey M, Paplinski A. General movement assessment by machine learning: Why is it so difficult? Journal of Medical Artificial Intelligence. 2019;**2**:15. Available from: https://jmai.amegroups.org/article/view/5058

[53] Rahmati H, Aamo OM, Stavdahl Ø, Dragon R, Adde L. Video-based early cerebral palsy prediction using motion segmentation. Annual International Conference of the IEEE Engineering in Medicine and Biology Society. 2014;**2014**:3779-3783. DOI: 10.1109/embc.2014.6944446

[54] Rahmati H, Martens H, Aamo OM, Stavdahl O, Stoen R, Adde L. Frequency analysis and feature reduction method for prediction of cerebral palsy in young infants. IEEE Transactions on Neural Systems and Rehabilitation Engineering. 2016;**24**(11):1225-1234. DOI: 10.1109/tnsre.2016.2539390

[55] Dai X, Wang S, Li H, Yue H, Min J. Image-Assisted Discrimination Method for Neurodevelopmental Disorders in Infants Based on Multi-Feature Fusion and Ensemble Learning. Brain Informatics. Cham: Springer International Publishing; 2019. p. 2019

[56] Nguyen-Thai B, Le V, Morgan C, Badawi N, Tran T, Venkatesh S. A Spatio-temporal attention-based model for infant movement assessment from videos. IEEE Journal of Biomedical and Health Informatics. 2021;**25**(10):3911-3920. DOI: 10.1109/JBHI.2021.3077957

[57] Kojovic N, Natraj S, Mohanty SP, Maillart T, Schaer M. Using 2D video-based pose estimation for automated prediction of autism spectrum disorders in young children. Scientific Reports. 2021;**11**(1):15069. DOI: 10.1038/s41598-021-94378-z

[58] Song C, Wang S, Chen M, Li H, Jia F, Zhao Y. A multimodal discrimination method for the response to name behavior of autistic children based on

human pose tracking and head pose estimation. Displays. 2023;**76**:102360. DOI: 10.1016/j.displa.2022.102360

[59] Zhou J, Smith BA. Infant reaching in the first year of life: A scoping review of typical development and examples of atypical development. Physical & Occupational Therapy in Pediatrics. 2022;**42**(1):80-98. DOI: 10.1080/01942638.2021.1921092

[60] Olsen JE, Brown NC, Eeles AL, Lee KJ, Anderson PJ, Cheong JL, et al. Trajectories of general movements from birth to term-equivalent age in infants born <30 weeks' gestation. Early Human Development. 2015;**91**(12):683-688. DOI: 10.1016/j.earlhumdev.2015.09.009

[61] Merino-Andrés J, Hidalgo-Robles Á, Pérez-Nombela S, Williams SA, Paleg G, Fernández-Rego FJ. Tool use for early detection of cerebral palsy: A survey of Spanish Pediatric physical therapists. Pediatric Physical Therapy. 2022;**34**(2):202-210. DOI: 10.1097/pep.0000000000000877

[62] Jardine LA, Mausling RM, Caldararo D, Colditz PW, Davies MW. Accelerometer measures in extremely preterm and or extremely low birth weight infants and association with abnormal general movements assessments at 28- and 32-weeks postmenstrual age. Early Human Development. 2022;**174**:105685. DOI: 10.1016/j.carlhumdcv.2022.105685

[63] Esterman E, Goyen TA, Jani P, Lowe G, Baird J, Maheshwari R, et al. Systemic postnatal corticosteroid use for the prevention of bronchopulmonary dysplasia and its relationship to early neurodevelopment in extremely preterm infants. World Journal of Pediatrics. 2023;**19**(6):586-594. DOI: 10.1007/s12519-023-00708-8

Chapter 9

Neonatal Anesthesia Neurotoxicity: A Review of the Evidence with Implications for Early Childhood Cleft and Craniofacial Surgery

Sheuli Chowdhury and Donald R. Laub Jr

Abstract

It is hypothesized that surgical anesthetic agents may be associated with damage to the early developing brain. There is animal evidence for anesthetic neurotoxicity, with basic science through behavioral studies demonstrating an increase in apoptosis and dendritic cell damage after exposure. However, these results have not been definitively translated to human studies. There continues to exist controversy in clinical research over whether early anesthetic exposure is associated with neurocognitive deficits, with many recent studies not supporting the theory of anesthetic drug-induced neurotoxicity in young children. There are three recent major human studies—the PANDA trial, the GAS trial, and the MASK trial—which contribute to our current perspective on anesthetic toxicity, overall suggesting that a single exposure for a healthy individual may be safe, but multiple exposures may have risk. Every surgery should contain a risk-benefit analysis to determine whether the advantages of an early procedure during a developmental phase justifies a potential neurotoxicity from the utilized anesthetics. We may need to re-evaluate the timing and number of stages of surgeries in our treatment protocols to account for these risks.

Keywords: neonatal, anesthesia, neurotoxicity, cognitive, neurodevelopment

1. Introduction

Millions of children worldwide each year undergo surgical, diagnostic, and therapeutic procedures that require pediatric anesthesia care. The only way that these can be safely done is by the implementation of safe and effective anesthesia practices. In our field of craniofacial surgery, the habilitation of children is only possible due to reliably safe and effective general anesthesia. Nevertheless, there persists concern that the administration of apparently uncomplicated general anesthetic in an otherwise healthy child, which is often readily used in adults, could lead to later neurocognitive deficits. A significant amount of research has gone into exploring these concerns;

however, the clinical significance of anesthetic neurotoxicity remains uncertain. It is incumbent on cleft and craniofacial surgeons, who commonly operate on infants during the neurocognitive developmental years, to strive for safety and lead this conversation.

Cleft and craniofacial surgeons are responsible for the care of children with craniofacial differences who require multiple staged procedures in their early childhood, and, thus, must assess whether the benefits of these procedures justify a potential, immeasurable anesthetic risk. We may need to re-evaluate the timing and number of stages of surgeries in our treatment protocols to account for these risks. An added pressure arises from the fact that this issue is discussed in the popular media, and worried parents may bring this as a concern to their surgical team. The evidence from animal studies for anesthetic neurotoxicity is concerning; however, larger human studies have conflictingly found less effect of anesthetic on neurocognitive development.

2. Animal studies

Animal research for the past decade has supported the hypothesis that the use of anesthetic agents during periods of rapid brain development, such as the neonatal years, are associated with increases in dendritic cell damage and neuroapoptosis in the central nervous system [1–7]. There have been a substantial number of articles implicating deficits in learning, memory and behavior in non-human species, particularly rats and primates [8–18]. Unfortunately, many commonly used anesthetic agents, including propofol, midazolam, and sevoflurane, have been implicated in neurocognitive development concerns.

Mechanistically, anesthetics tend to work on GABA and NMDA receptors. For instance, propofol and sevoflurane bind to GABA-A receptors to enhance inhibitory GABA effects. Sevoflurane and ketamine antagonize NMDA receptors. The agents' involvement in these and other pathways may incidentally cause cognitive impairment. For instance, sevoflurane has been implicated in the ubiquitination-proteasome pathway [10]. Increasing doses of propofol, midazolam, isoflurane, and ketamine have all been associated with activating caspase-3, which is a marker of

Study	Year	Model	Outcome measures	Findings
Song et al.	2019	Mouse	ABGs, behavioral studies, and RNA sequencing	There are differentially expressed genes in the hippocampus following multiple anesthetic exposures, inducing social behavior disorders.
Cattano et al.	2008	Mouse	Quantitative activated caspase-3 levels following propofol exposure	Propofol triggers neuroapoptosis in the developing mouse brain.
Brambrink et al.	2010	Rhesus monkey	Quantitative activated caspase 3-stained neurons following isoflurane exposure	Exposing infant rhesus macaques to five hours of anesthetic is associated with a 13-fold increased rate of neuroapoptosis.
Brambrink et al.	2012	Rhesus monkey	Location of apoptosis within the brain following exposure	Oligodendrocytes were selectively vulnerable for apoptosis following anesthetic exposure in infant rhesus macaques.

Study	Year	Model	Outcome measures	Findings
Jevtovic-Todorovic et al.	2003	Rat	ABGs, activated caspase-3 levels, electrophysiological studies, behavioral studies	Exposure to anesthesia resulted in lasting deficits in hippocampal, anterior thalamic nuclei, mammillary bodies, and retrosplenial cortex synaptic function, mediated by GABA and NDMA
Creeley et al.	2013	Rhesus monkey	Activated caspase-3 levels as a measure of apoptotic degeneration	Five hours of propofol exposure was associated with neuronal and oligodendrocyte apoptosis.
Coleman et al.	2017	Rhesus monkey	Behavioral studies	Following multiple isoflurane exposures, monkeys had reflex deficits and increased anxiety. This was not seen after single exposure.
Raper et al.	2015, 2018	Rhesus monkey	Behavioral studies	Following multiple sevoflurane exposures, monkeys had a higher frequency of anxiety-related behaviors and emotional reactivity.

Table 1.
Noteworthy animal anesthetic risk studies.

neuroapoptosis. Gene expression, using RNA sequencing, is also impacted following multiple anesthetic exposures. Studies have isolated specific neural locations and cell types affected by anesthetic exposure, finding the hippocampus, anterior thalamic nuclei, mammillary bodies, retrosplenial cortex, and oligodendrocytes to be particularly susceptible [6]. **Table 1** summarizes findings from recent animal studies.

These well-documented findings serve as the source for significant concern when translating the potential neurocognitive effects of early anesthetic exposure to human patients.

3. Human studies

On the other hand, studies in humans are less clear regarding neonatal toxicity. In comparison to animal studies, human studies are obviously limited by ethical considerations. There are three recent, major prospective human trials on pediatric anesthesia. The Pediatric Anesthesia & Neurodevelopment Assessment (PANDA) trial was a large, multicenter, sibling-matched cohort study from Columbia University conducted between 2009 and 2015 [19]. They compared healthy siblings where one had a single anesthesia exposure during an inguinal hernia surgery prior to the age of three, and the other did not. The primary outcome of intelligence quotient (IQ) and secondary cognitive assessments were evaluated years later, between participant ages of eight and fifteen, to allow time for neurocognitive development. The study found no significant difference in IQ between the two siblings. They also did not find any statistically significant differences in secondary outcomes, including memory, attention, visuospatial function, adaptive behavior, executive function, and verbal fluency. Limitations of this study include lack of analysis on repeated neonatal anesthesia exposure and female participants.

The general anesthesia vs. awake-regional anesthesia (GAS) study recruited infants from 2007 to 2013 as an international collaboration of institutions from Australia, the United States, Canada, Italy, the United Kingdom, New Zealand, and the Netherlands [20]. The investigators performed an assessor-blinded, randomized control clinical trial on infants under 60 weeks old who were born after 26 weeks of gestation and scheduled to undergo inguinal hernia repair. The participants were randomly assigned to receive either general anesthesia with sevoflurane or regional spinal anesthesia with bupivacaine or levobupivacaine. Five year follow ups were performed with the Wechsler Preschool and Primary Scale of Intelligence Full Scale Intelligence Quotient (WPPSI-III FSIQ) as a measure of neurocognitive function. They found that, following the median duration of about 1 hour of anesthesia exposure in the first 60 weeks of life, there were no significant difference in IQ and neurodevelopmental outcomes in children after 5 years. Similarly to the prior study, the GAS study was limited by its lack of analysis on female children and children with repeated anesthesia exposures.

Finally, the Mayo Anesthesia Safety in Kids (MASK) trial from the Mayo Clinic recruited children who were unexposed, singly exposed, or multiply exposed to anesthesia prior to the age of three between 1994 and 2007 [21]. They then used the Wechsler Abbreviated Scale of Intelligence (WASI) scale to evaluate IQ and other measures of neurocognitive development between the ages of 8–12 and 15–20. They found that any amount of exposure to anesthesia did not have an association with significant differences of IQ as the primary outcome. However, multiple anesthesia exposures may be associated with reduction of secondary outcomes of processing speed, fine motor coordination, and parent reported difficulties with behavior and reading. A strength of this study is its evaluation of the effect of repeated exposures; however, limitations include an inability to account for inherent differences that may result in patients requiring multiple early procedures, varied anesthetic types, and an uncontrolled variable of half of the participants having anesthetic exposure after the age of three (**Table 2**).

Study	Publication year	Recruitment location	Study size	Findings
PANDA	2016	USA	105 paired siblings	Following a single anesthetic exposure, there was no significant difference in IQ, memory, attention, visuospatial function, adaptive behavior, executive function, and verbal fluency between two siblings.
GAS	2019	Australia, Italy, USA, UK, Canada, Netherlands, and New Zealand	205 children with regional anesthetic vs. 242 general	Following a median of one 1 of single anesthetic exposure in the first 60 weeks of life, there were no significant difference in IQ or neurocognitive development outcomes in children.
MASK	2018	USA	997 children	Any amount of exposure to anesthesia (single or repeated) was not associated with IQ differences. However, multiple exposures may be associated with reduction of processing speed, fine motor coordination, and parent reported difficulties with behavior and reading.

Table 2.
Noteworthy human anesthetic risk trials.

There are numerous smaller human studies that have corroborated the theory that neonatal anesthesia has minimal effects on neurocognitive development [22, 23]. However, the data is mixed. The current findings remain contradictory, with some evidence also suggesting that there may exist small differences in neurocognitive development that remain critical to be explored [3, 24, 25]. Additionally, along with the MASK trial, there are other studies supporting the theory that repeated exposure may be associated with worse long-term cognitive outcomes [26–28].

4. Application to neonatal surgery

The above human studies focused on otherwise healthy children with surgeries that do not necessarily reflect an underlying condition that may complicate the neurocognitive development. Children born with cleft lips and palate provide an interesting population of relatively healthy children that typically require multiple exposures to anesthesia at a young age.

Pediatric craniofacial surgeons typically treat children with cleft lip and cleft palate using treatment protocols that require at least two surgeries, or multiple anesthetic exposures, during infancy. There is critical evidence supporting the theory that these surgeries are time-sensitive; specifically, palate repair will provide a superior speech outcome if it is performed before the critical period of language acquisition. There are decades of level III evidence case series that address this argument. In 1982, Dorf and Curtin found that children who received a palate repair after the age of 1 year had a 90% incidence of compensatory articulations, whereas those who had the repair prior to the 12 months of age had a less than 5% incidence of compensatory articulations [29]. A similar finding was discovered by Chapman and Hardin in the same year of a 90% incidence of compensatory articulations for late palate repairs [30].

In 2000, Kirschner et al. compared children undergoing Furlow palatoplasties prior to 7 months of age and after, and they found no significant difference in speech scores, velopharyngeal incompetence, and rate of secondary pharyngoplasty [31]. In 2008, Chapman et al. compared lexical outcomes in a level II multicenter prospective series for children undergoing palatal surgery. They discovered that those operated on under the age of 11 months with less preoperative lexical ability ultimately had better speech outcomes than those with better preoperative lexical ability with their surgery at a mean age of 15 months [32]. There are additional recent studies supporting equivalent or superior outcomes for cleft lip repair in children younger than 3 months of age [33, 34]. All these studies show that there may be lexical benefits to early operative intervention that must be weighed against the theoretical risk of early anesthetic exposure.

The Timing for Primary Surgery (TOPS) trial, recently published in 2023, is a multicenter, randomized controlled trial conducted across Brazil, Denmark, Norway, Sweden, and the UK [35]. Infants were assigned to receive surgery at either 6 months or 12 months of age. They found that those with earlier surgeries had significantly lower incidence of velopharyngeal insufficiency by 5 years of age. At 1 year old, canonical babbling, hearing sensitivity, and middle-ear function were better in children with earlier repair, however this difference became insignificant by 5 years of age. Notably, early repair was more significantly associated with maxillary arch constriction, though other technical outcomes were similar. These findings across the above studies may indicate persuasive support for early operative intervention, which should be weighed against potential risks.

Craniofacial surgeons also frequently refer children for perioperative diagnostic imaging procedures that require anesthesia. The same trepidations applied to surgical anesthesia exposure risk should be considered for diagnostic and planning imaging studies on young children, who often circumstantially require general anesthesia to complete required studies. Is there a theoretical benefit to limiting the number of preoperative studies or operative stages to deliver a comparative effective care while minimizing risks? There are few studies that explore this. Conrad et al. retrospectively reviewed children with cleft palates and found no association between number of surgeries and academic ability but did find a negative association with social involvement [36]. Clausen et al. compared academic scores of children with cleft lip or cleft palate or both, and found that cleft type affected academic outcomes, but number of surgeries did not, though they acknowledged that this latter finding was limited and ambiguous [37].

While we continue to research for more definitive answers to this dilemma, neonatal and pediatric surgeons should familiarize themselves with this issue and develop answers to questions from parents seeking reassurance and better understanding. Some pediatric surgeries (including lower extremity procedures, inguinal hernia repairs, circumcision, etc.) can be safely and efficiently conducted under a regional anesthetic technique such as spinal anesthesia with much less presumed neurocognitive risk. Multiple studies have shown that spinal anesthesia is effective and safe with respect to neurological risk and should be explored if appropriate [38–40]. However, this is not necessarily possible with all surgeries, particularly cleft and craniofacial procedures. These surgeries and the required anesthesia for a safe operation should not be withheld from children in need.

The clear next question is, if we accept that there may be an anesthetic neurocognitive risk for young children, particularly in the incidence of multiple exposures, what can be done to mitigate this effect on our cleft and craniofacial patients who cannot rely on spinal or local anesthesia due to the location of the operation? Shorter operations may mitigate risk, so surgical technique could be modified to prioritize brevity of anesthetic exposure. Postoperatively, patients may benefit from focused developmental training in implicated cognitive fields, including fine motor coordination, behavior, and reading. Further research should be done on molecular and animal models to compare the different anesthetics and determine if certain agents have less neurodegenerative impact. One recent study associated propofol specifically with less effect on neurocognition [41]. There is certainly room for more exploration of this field.

5. Conclusion

Currently, the evidence for neonatal anesthetic toxicity is not yet definitive on whether recommendations should be made regarding age at or number of procedures. Certainly, multiple large studies seem to suggest that it may be safe to perform anesthesia on infants in the neurodevelopmental period; however, there does seem to be a contradiction between human and animal models [42]. The surgeon must weigh a recommendation to delay or limit these procedures against the benefits of early surgical repair. In the field of craniofacial surgery, could there be a reduced risk of neurocognitive toxicity by changing a surgical protocol to one of shorter, later, or fewer staged repairs, or would that too significantly imbalance the scale toward poorer patient outcomes? [43] Could patients at risk benefit from focused neurodevelopmental training postoperatively? Potential risks and benefits should continue to be investigated to promote the long-term safety of our young patient population. Surgeons of all surgical subspecialties should be aware of the concerns of anesthesiologists, pediatricians, and the public regarding potential neurotoxicity of general anesthetics, and they should be cognizant of the limitations of the current evidence.

Conflict of interest

The authors declare no conflict of interest.

Author details

Sheuli Chowdhury* and Donald R. Laub Jr
University of Vermont Medical Center, Burlington, Vermont,
United States of America

*Address all correspondence to: sheuli.chowdhury@uvmhealth.org

References

[1] Song SY, Meng XW, Xia Z, Liu H, Zhang J, Chen QC, et al. Cognitive impairment and transcriptomic profile in hippocampus of young mice after multiple neonatal exposures to sevoflurane. Aging (Albany NY). 2019;**11**(19):8386-8417. DOI: 10.18632/aging.102326. Epub 2019 Oct 3

[2] Cattano D, Young C, Straiko MM, Olney J. Subanesthetic doses of propofol induce neuroapoptosis in the infant mouse brain. Anesthesia and Analgesia. 2008;**106**:1712-1714

[3] Block RI, Thomas JJ, Bayman EO, Choi JY, Kimble KK, Todd MM. Are anesthesia and surgery during infancy associated with altered academic performance during childhood? Anesthesiology. 2012;**117**:494-503

[4] Brambrink AM, Evers AS, Avidan MS, Farber NB, Smith DJ, Zhang X, et al. Isoflurane-induced neuroapoptosis in the neonatal rhesus macaque brain. Anesthesiology. 2010;**112**:834-841

[5] Brambrink AM, Back SA, Riddle A, Gong X, Moravec MD, Dissen GA, et al. Isoflurane-induced apoptosis of oligodendrocytes in the neonatal primate brain. Annals of Neurology. 2012;**72**:525-535

[6] Jevtovic-Todorovic V, Hartman RE, Izumi Y, Benshoff ND, Dikranian K, Zorumski CF, et al. Early exposure to common anesthetic agents causes widespread neurodegeneration in the developing rat brain and persistent learning deficits. The Journal of Neuroscience. 2003;**23**:876-892

[7] Creeley C, Dikranian K, Dissen G, Martin L, Olney J, Brambrink A. Propofol-induced apoptosis of neurons and oligodendrocytes in fetal and neonatal rhesus macaque brain. British Journal of Anesthesia. 2013;**110**(Suppl. 1):i29-i38

[8] Shen X, Liu Y, Xu S, Zhao Q, Guo X, Shen R, et al. Early life exposure to sevoflurane impairs adulthood spatial memory in the rat. Neurotoxicology. 2013;**39**:45-56. DOI: 10.1016/j.neuro.2013.08.007. Epub 2013 Aug 27

[9] Shen X, Dong Y, Xu Z, Wang H, Miao C, Soriano SG, et al. Selective anesthesia-induced neuroinflammation in developing mouse brain and cognitive impairment. Anesthesiology. 2013;**118**:502-515

[10] Lu H, Liufu N, Dong Y, Xu G, Zhang Y, Shu L, et al. Sevoflurane acts on ubiquitination-proteasome pathway to reduce postsynaptic density 95 protein levels in young mice. Anesthesiology. 2017;**127**(6):961-975. DOI: 10.1097/ALN.0000000000001889

[11] Jin LH, Song YY, Shen Y, Ji W, Zhang MZ. Post-exposure exercise fails to ameliorate memory impairment induced by propofol and ketamine in developing rats. Medical Science Monitor. 2016;**22**:1038-1046. DOI: 10.12659/msm.895443

[12] Raper J, Alvarado MC, Murphy KL, Baxter MG. Multiple anesthetic exposure in infant monkeys alters emotional reactivity to an acute stressor. Anesthesiology. 2015;**123**(5):1084-1092. DOI: 10.1097/ALN.0000000000000851

[13] Alvarado MC, Murphy KL, Baxter MG. Visual recognition memory is impaired in rhesus monkeys repeatedly exposed to sevoflurane in infancy. British Journal of Anaesthesia.

2017;**119**(3):517-523. DOI: 10.1093/bja/aew473

[14] Coleman K, Robertson ND, Dissen GA, Neuringer MD, Martin LD, Cuzon Carlson VC, et al. Isoflurane anesthesia has long-term consequences on motor and behavioral development in infant rhesus macaques. Anesthesiology. 2017;**126**(1):74-84. DOI: 10.1097/ALN.0000000000001383

[15] Raper J, De Biasio JC, Murphy KL, Alvarado MC, Baxter MG. Persistent alteration in behavioural reactivity to a mild social stressor in rhesus monkeys repeatedly exposed to sevoflurane in infancy. British Journal of Anaesthesia. 2018;**120**(4):761-767. DOI: 10.1016/j.bja.2018.01.014. Epub 2018 Mar 1

[16] Paule MG, Li M, Allen RR, Liu F, Zou X, Hotchkiss C, et al. Ketamine anesthesia during the first week of life can cause long-lasting cognitive deficits in rhesus monkeys. Neurotoxicology and Teratology. 2011;**33**:220-230

[17] Takaenoki Y, Satoh Y, Araki Y, Kodama M, Yonamine R, Yufune S, et al. Neonatal exposure to sevoflurane in mice causes deficits in maternal behavior later in adulthood. Anesthesiology. 2014;**120**:403-415

[18] Neudecker V, Perez-Zoghbi JF, Martin LD, Dissen GA, Grafe MR, Brambrink AM. Astrogliosis in juvenile non-human primates 2 years after infant anaesthesia exposure. British Journal of Anaesthesia. 2021;**127**(3):447-457. DOI: 10.1016/j.bja.2021.04.034. Epub 2021 Jul 13

[19] Sun LS, Li G, Miller TL, Salorio C, Byrne MW, Bellinger DC, et al. Association between a single general anesthesia exposure before age 36 months and neurocognitive outcomes in later childhood. Journal of the American Medical Association. 2016;**315**(21):2312-2320. DOI: 10.1001/jama.2016.6967

[20] ME MC, de Graaff JC, Dorris L, Disma N, Withington D, Bell G, et al. Neurodevelopmental outcome at 5 years of age after general anaesthesia or awake-regional anaesthesia in infancy (GAS): An international, multicentre, randomised, controlled equivalence trial. Lancet. 2019;**393**(10172):664-677. DOI: 10.1016/S0140-6736(18)32485-1. Epub 2019 Feb 14. Erratum in: Lancet. 2019 Aug 24;394(10199):638. DOI: 10.1016/S0140-6736(19)31958-0

[21] Warner DO, Zaccariello MJ, Katusic SK, Schroeder DR, Hanson AC, Schulte PJ, et al. Neuropsychological and behavioral outcomes after exposure of young children to procedures requiring general anesthesia: The mayo anesthesia safety in kids (MASK) study. Anesthesiology. 2018;**129**(1):89-105. DOI: 10.1097/ALN.0000000000002232

[22] Hansen TG, Pedersen JK, Henneberg SW, Pedersen DA, Murray JC, Morton NS, et al. Academic performance in adolescence after inguinal hernia repair in infancy: A nationwide cohort study. Anesthesiology. 2011;**114**(5):1076-1085. DOI: 10.1097/ALN.0b013e31820e77a0

[23] O'Leary JD, Janus M, Duku E, Wijeysundera DN, To T, Li P, et al. Influence of surgical procedures and general anesthesia on child development before primary school entry among matched sibling pairs. JAMA Pediatrics. 2019;**173**(1):29-36. DOI: 10.1001/jamapediatrics.2018.3662

[24] Glatz P, Sandin RH, Pedersen NL, Bonamy AK, Eriksson LI, Granath F. Association of anesthesia and surgery during childhood with long-term academic performance. JAMA Pediatrics. 2017;**171**(1):e163470. DOI: 10.1001/jamapediatrics.2016.3470. Epub 2017 Jan 2

[25] de Heer IJ, Tiemeier H, Hoeks SE, Weber F. Intelligence quotient scores at the age of 6 years in children anaesthetised before the age of 5 years. Anaesthesia. 2017;**72**(1):57-62. DOI: 10.1111/anae.13687. Epub 2016 Sep 26

[26] Flick RP, Katusic SK, Colligan RC, Wilder RT, Voigt RG, Olson MD, et al. Cognitive and behavioral outcomes after early exposure to anesthesia and surgery. Pediatrics. 2011;**128**:e1053-e1061

[27] Sprung J, Flick RP, Katusic SK, Colligan RC, Barbaresi WJ, Bojanić K, et al. Attention-deficit/hyperactivity disorder after early exposure to procedures requiring general anesthesia. Mayo Clinic Proceedings. 2012;**87**(2):120-129. DOI: 10.1016/j.mayocp.2011.11.008

[28] Wilder RT, Flick RP, Sprung J, Katusic SK, Barbaresi WJ, Mickelson C, et al. Early exposure to anesthesia and learning disabilities in a population-based birth cohort. Anesthesiology. 2009;**110**:796-804

[29] Dorf DS, Curtin JW. Early cleft repair and speech outcome. Plastic and Reconstructive Surgery. 1982;**70**:74-79

[30] Chapman KL, Hardin-Jones MA. Phonetic and phonological skills of two-year-olds with cleft palate. The Cleft Palate-Craniofacial Journal. 1992;**29**:435-443

[31] Kirschner RE, Randall P, Wang P, Jawad AF, Duran M, Huang K, et al. Cleft palate repair at 3-7 months of age. Plastic and Reconstructive Surgery. 2000;**105**(6):2127-2137

[32] Chapman KL, Hardin-Jones MA, Goldstein JA, Halter KA, Havlik RJ, Schulte J. Timing of palatal surgery and speech outcome. The Cleft Palate-Craniofacial Journal. 2008;**45**(3):297-308

[33] Kondra K, Stanton E, Jimenez C, Ngo K, Wlodarczyk J, Jacob L, et al. Rethinking the rule of 10s: Early cleft lip repair improves weight gain. The Cleft Palate-Craniofacial Journal. 2023;**60**(3):306-312. DOI: 10.1177/10556656211062042. Epub 2021 Dec 6

[34] Wlodarczyk JR, Wolfswinkel EM, Liu A, Fahradyan A, Higuchi E, Goel P, et al. Early cleft lip repair: Demonstrating efficacy in the first 100 patients. Plastic and Reconstructive Surgery. 2022;**150**(5):1073-1080. DOI: 10.1097/PRS.0000000000009634. Epub 2022 Aug 24

[35] Gamble C, Persson C, Willadsen E, Albery L, Soegaard Andersen H, Zattoni Antoneli M, et al. TOPS study group. Timing of primary surgery for cleft palate. The New England Journal of Medicine. 2023;**389**(9):795-807. DOI: 10.1056/NEJMoa2215162

[36] Conrad AL, Albert M, Crerand CE, Crilly Bellucci C, Heppner CE, Sheikh F, et al. Retrospective evaluation of number of surgeries and parent ratings of academic and behavioral functioning among children with isolated oral clefts. The Cleft Palate-Craniofacial Journal. 2021;**58**(10):1294-1303. DOI: 10.1177/1055665620982807. Epub 2020 Dec 30

[37] Clausen NG, Pedersen DA, Pedersen JK, Møllcr SE, Grosen D, Wehby GL, et al. Oral clefts and academic performance in adolescence: The impact of anesthesia-related neurotoxicity, timing of surgery, and type of oral clefts. The Cleft Palate-Craniofacial Journal. 2017;**54**(4):371-380. DOI: 10.1597/15-185. Epub 2016 Apr 4

[38] Williams RK, Adams DC, Aladjem EV, Kreutz JM, Sartorelli KH, Vane DW, et al. The safety and efficacy

of spinal anesthesia for surgery in infants: The Vermont Infant Spinal Registry. Anesthesia and Analgesia. 2006;**102**(1):67-71

[39] Hamurtekin E, Fitzsimmons BL, Shubayev VI, Grafe MR, Deumens R, Yaksh TL, et al. Evaluation of spinal toxicity and long-term spinal reflex function after intrathecal levobupivaciane in the neonatal rat. Anesthesiology. 2013;**119**:142-155

[40] Yahalom B, Athiraman U, Soriano SG, Zurakowski D, Carpino EA, Corfas G, et al. Spinal anesthesia in infant rats: Development of a model and assessment of neurologic outcomes. Anesthesiology. 2011;**114**(6):1325-1335

[41] Dandemmanavar V, Vikas KN, Vinay R, Bandyopadhyay S, Gakhar H, Dey A. The impact of anesthetic agents on neurocognitive outcomes in pediatric patients. Journal of Neonatal Surgery. 2025;**14**(10s):153-161

[42] Shao LJ, Zou Y, Xue FS. Anesthesia-induced developmental neurotoxicity in children: Past, present, and future. Chinese Medical Journal. 2019;**132**(16):1990-1992. DOI: 10.1097/CM9.0000000000000377

[43] Laub DR Jr, Williams RK. Neonatal anesthesia neurotoxicity: A review for cleft and craniofacial surgeons. The Cleft Palate-Craniofacial Journal. 2015;**52**(4):494-498. DOI: 10.1597/14-126. Epub 2014 Jun 18